Caregivers of Persons Living with HIV/AIDS in Kenya

An Ecological Perspective

Published by:
Adonis & Abbey Publishers Ltd
P. O. Box 43418
London, United Kingdom
SE11 4XZ

Nigeria
Adonis & Abbey Publishing Co
P.O. Box 10546
Abuja, Nigeria
Tel: +234 (0)8165970458

http://www.adonis-abbey.com
Email: editor@adonis-abbey.com

First Edition, December 2011

British Library Cataloguing-in-Publication Data
A catalogue record for this book is available from the British Library

ISBN: 9781906704827

Layout Artist, Jan B. Mwesigwa, www.janmwesigwa.com

Printed and bound in Great Britain

Caregivers of Persons Living with HIV/AIDS in Kenya

An Ecological Perspective

Charnetta Gadling-Cole
Sandra Edmonds Crewe
Mildred C. Joyner

Foreword by Grace Jepkemboi

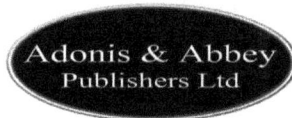

Adonis & Abbey
Publishers Ltd

CONTENTS

List of Tables and Figures

FOREWORD

During the early years of the past century, many people in Africa and other parts of the world could not even perceive HIV/AIDS and its impact in the world. Thus, a book purporting to be a "guide to caregivers for persons living with HIV/AIDS" would have been an anachronism. The traditional family was a self-contained economic and social unit. Families desired and bore many children, and the family included grandparents, parents, uncles, aunts, and cousins. It was a communal center with parents at the hub, responsible for the care of their children and instilling societal values. Then the famous African proverb, "It takes a village to raise a child," adequately described Africa and its solid form of communal care.

Today, the continent, communities, and families are different. The changes that have occurred over the past quarter of a century are profound. The strong tightly knit and intricate African society has slowly been eroded by several factors, including HIV/AIDS. Like the rest of the continent, Kenya has felt the gruesome effects of HIV/AIDS. The first case of HIV was diagnosed in Kenya in 1985. Since then, HIV/AIDS has escalated from a rare disease to an epidemic, then a pandemic. According to the most recent Kenya Demographic and Health Survey (KDHS, 2008-2009), 1.6- 1.9 million of the 38.6 million Kenyan residents is living with HIV/AIDS, and 2.4 million children are orphaned by AIDS. The adult HIV prevalence in Kenya has now stabilized to around 6.3 percent.

HIV/AIDS is overwhelming the traditional systems of care. HIV prevalence is nearly two times higher among adult women compared to men. Thus, women and young adults, who are the most productive and economic engines as well as primary caregivers in the society, are being slowly eliminated by HIV/AIDS. Therefore, society is revisiting its mode of care. The two forms of care that have emerged as a result of AIDS are grandparents raising grandchildren and home-based care for people living with HIV/AIDS. Because of the rising cost of care and lack of enough room at the health care units in Kenya, many people living with HIV/AIDS, are often sent home to be cared for by surviving spouses and relatives. Families caring for their loved ones affected by AIDS also encounter emotional, financial, moral, and social challenges. Hence, the new face of care giving in Kenya needs a lot of professional support.

For this reason, the appearance of a book, *"Caregiver for Persons Living with HIV/AIDS in Kenya: An Ecological perspective,"* is most welcome. This book is a thoughtful guide to more productive relationships between caregivers and their loved ones living with HIV/AIDS. It begins with the premise that caregivers in Kenya did not choose their destiny, and further exposes the trials, tribulations, and challenges those caregivers encounter as they try to provide the best care they can afford for their loved ones.

This book makes clear that home-based care in Kenya is a better option of care for families caring for loved ones living with HIV/AIDS. The framework for home-based care and its' principles are discussed. The authors describe the home-based needs at various levels. The text is grounded on sound research and adequate theoretical perspectives used in social work. The authors also make several practical recommendations for care giving based on the perspectives of caregivers of people living with HIV/AIDS.

This book also presents a multidisciplinary approach to care for people living with AIDS in Kenya. The authors emphasize the role of churches and other faith based organizations in working with care givers to provide social, moral and spiritual support. They also highlight the important role of International Social Work; Council on Social Work Education, International Federation of Social Workers, and the International Association of Schools of Social Work in joining hands and providing expertise and grounded research to provide better and appropriate practices for caregivers of HIV/AIDs patients.

It is important to note that though a lot of attention has been placed on the efforts to find the cure for HIV/AIDS, very little emphasis and resources have been placed on home-based care for the patients. This book fills a large share of that void. It helps change the landscape by providing a tool in the hands of caregivers to enable them to provide better care to their affected loved ones. I am pleased that the editors and contributors are sharing their ground breaking research and their recommendations with the caregivers of HIV/AIDS patients, students of social work, social workers, and professionals in the field all over the world.

Dr. Grace Jepkemboi
University of Alabama at Birmingham

PREFACE AND ACKNOWLEDGEMENTS

The work of caregiving for individuals, families, and communities with HIV and AIDS falls heavily on volunteers and members of the weakened extended family network. They are joined by churches, FBOs, and NGOs to fill the gaps in familial networks. As social workers, we are pleased to offer a transnational hand in addressing the important family work to be done. As African American women, we understand the dynamics of oppression, gender inequality, and poverty. Equally important is our understanding of the unique roles of the formal and informal care systems.

Using the ecological perspective, we present the voices of the caregivers in a way that recognizes that people and environment are one. According to Mandella (1999), a person with Ubuntu is open and available to others, affirming of others, does not feel threatened that others are able and good, for he or she has a proper self-assurance that comes from knowing that he or she belongs in a greater whole and is diminished when others are humiliated or diminished, when others are tortured or oppressed. Similarly, Prof. Wangari Maathai, a former Kenyan Government Minister and the first African woman to win a Nobel Prize states "All of us have a God in us, and that God is the spirit that unites all life, everything that is on this planet."

Dr. Inabel Burns Lindsay, founding Dean of the Howard University School of Social Work, developed a social work curriculum that emphasized the importance of culture in delivering effective services to vulnerable populations. Lindsay's socio-cultural perspective has evolved today to what many social work practitioners refer to as cultural competence. She recognized that working with individuals would not bring about change without change in the mezzo and macro systems in society. Her ecological approach differed somewhat from those of social work educators and practitioners, who addressed culture but did not link their understanding of culture directly with socioeconomic power differentials, class, or institutional racism. Additionally, Dr. Lindsay emphasized the importance of a transnational application of the socio cultural perspective for effective social work practice (Brown, Gourdine & Crewe, 2011; Crewe, Gourdine, & Brown, 2007); Gourdine, Crewe & Brown, (2008). All three authors of this book have also been exposed to the teachings of Dr. Lindsay through their study at Howard University and this book reflects the influence of her ideology.

In presenting the voices of caregivers, there is a strong Ubuntu presence as the authors explore the challenges related to women and children; financial hardships; food, clothing, shelter and transportation; widowhood; stigmatization and discrimination; employment; safety; treatment; training and support; and advocacy.

The caregivers and organizations participating in this research are owed a tremendous debt of gratitude. Their voices are critical to the continuing effort to improve the quality of life of individuals, families, and communities infected and affected by HIV and AIDS.

Sandra Edmonds Crewe, Ph.D., MSW,ACSW
Howard University School of Social Work

The authors would like to acknowledge Yvonne Holmes, Executive Director, Higher Ground Outreach, Decatur, Georgia for sponsoring and coordinating the caregiver research in Nairobi, Kenya.

Chapter 1

HISTORICAL OVERVIEW AND BACKGROUND

"Community and faith-based organizations have a critical role to play in the provision of HIV/AIDS prevention, care, and treatment. They possess an extensive geographic reach and a well-developed infrastructure in the developing world. This, in addition to their unmatched staying power, makes them an invaluable asset in the fight against the HIV/AIDS pandemic."
(PEPFAR, 2006)

Profile of Kenya

The Republic of Kenya is situated on the equator on Africa's east coast. Kenya has been described as "the cradle of humanity" because some of the earliest evidence of our ancestors were found there. Its scenic beauty and abundant wildlife also makes Kenya one of Africa's major safari destinations and accounts for tourism being the leading foreign currency earner followed by horticulture and tea. The capital of Kenya is Nairobi. The life expectancy of Kenyans is 56 years for men and 57 years for women. Poverty, high unemployment, and crime are among its most pressing challenges, and most Kenyans live below the poverty level of $1 per day (BBS, 2011).

Kenya has a very diverse population that includes three of Africa's major sociolinguistic groups: Bantu (67%), Nilotic (30%), and Cushitic (3%). Kenyans are deeply religious. About 80% of Kenyans are Christian, 11% are Muslim, and the remainder follow traditional African religions or other faiths. Most city residents retain links with their rural, extended families and leave the city periodically to help work on the family farm. About 75% of the work force is engaged in agriculture, mainly as subsistence farm-

1

ers. The national motto of Kenya is *Harambee*, meaning "pull together." In that spirit, volunteers in hundreds of communities build schools, clinics, and other facilities each year and collect funds to send students abroad (US State Department, 2011).

Although this book focuses on HIV/AIDS and caregivers, it is important to present a profile of the country that acknowledges its strengths and assets as well. This knowledge helps to place the findings of the research within context.

History of HIV and AIDS

HIV/AIDS is now recognized as a global health crisis. HIV has generated substantial attention and controversy with the main questions being, "Where did the virus come from? And, how did it spread to all corners of the earth?" There are a number of theories that some would say range from absurd to plausible – the debate continues. Common theories are the claim that AIDS is "divine punishment to a sinful generation" and the conspiracy theory that "HIV was deliberately created in a laboratory and then introduced into the African population" (Muraah & Kiarie, 2001).

In the early 1980s, doctors started frequently seeing a rare illness in homosexual men in San Francisco and New York. Tests performed on these men revealed that their immune system was greatly weakened; however, the cause could not be identified. The doctors hypothesized that a new infectious organism was damaging the immune system. By 1982, researches were convinced that this was not just a homosexual disease. The same year the disease received its current name, Acquired Immuno Deficiency Syndrome: AIDS (Muraah & Kiarie, 2001).

Cichocki (2009) asserts that the history of HIV is filled with "triumphs and failures; living and death" (pg 1). In July of 1981, the New York Times reported an outbreak of a rare form of cancer among gay men in New York and California. It was referred to as the "gay cancer" but was later identified as Kaposi's Sarcoma, a disease that later became the face of HIV/AIDS. Emergency rooms in New York City began to see a large number of seemingly healthy young men with fevers, flu-like symptoms, and a rare pneumonia called Pneumocystis. This was the beginning of what has become the biggest health care pandemic in modern history. The following table provides a comprehensive societal timeline of HIV/AIDS.

Figure 1:   Maps of Kenya

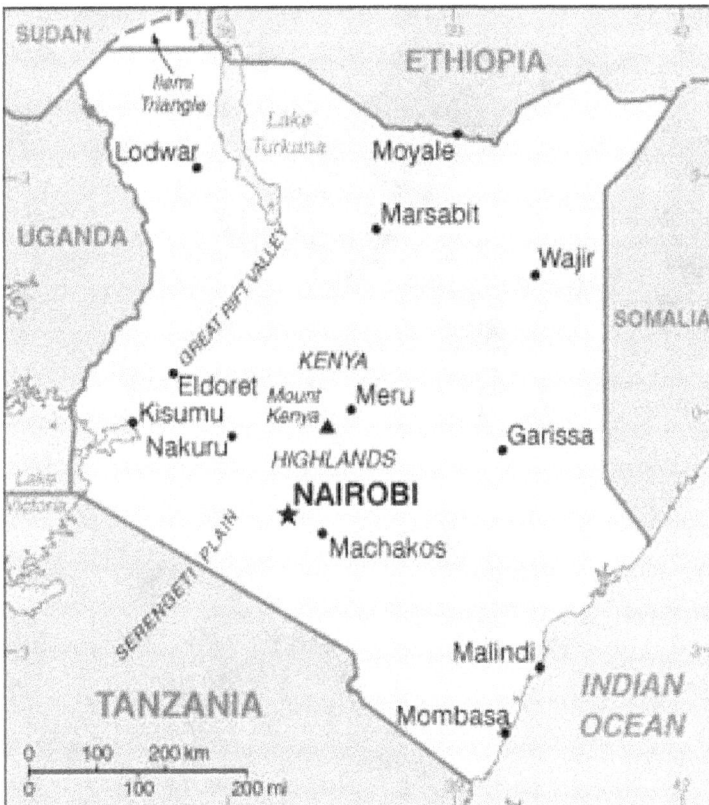

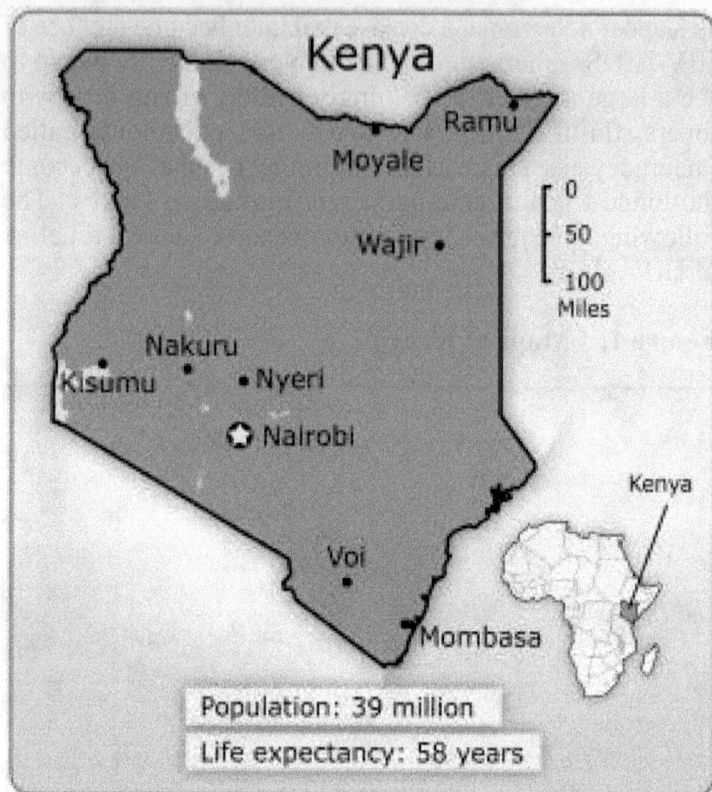

Table 1: Comprehensive Societal Timeline of HIV/AIDS

1959 While we talk about HIV/AIDS being 25 years old, in actuality it is believed that the syndrome has been around far longer. In 1959, a man residing in Africa died of a mysterious illness. Only decades later after examining some blood samples taken from that man was it confirmed that he actually died from complications related to an HIV infection.

1981 1981 saw the emergence of Kaposi's Sarcoma and Pneumocystis among gay men in New York and California. When the Centers for Disease Control reported the new outbreak, they called it "GRID" (gay-related immune deficiency), stigmatizing the gay community as carriers of this deadly disease. However, cases started to be seen in heterosexuals, drug addicts, and people who received blood transfusions, proving the syndrome knew no boundaries.

1983 Researchers at the Pasteur Institute in France isolate a retrovirus that they believe is related to the outbreak of HIV/AIDS. Thirty-three countries around the world have confirmed cases of the disease that was once limited to New York and California. Controversy arises a year later when the US government announces their scientist, Dr. Robert Gallo isolates a retrovirus HTLV-III, that he too claims is responsible for AIDS. Two years later, it is confirmed that HTLV-III and the Pasteur retrovirus are indeed the same virus, yet Gallo is still credited with its discovery. An international committee of scientists renames the virus HIV.

1984 A Canadian flight attendant, nicknamed "patient zero" dies of AIDS. Because of his sexual connection to several of the first victims of HIV/AIDS, it is believed that he is responsible for introducing the virus into the general population.
*8000 confirmed cases in the US *3700 confirmed deaths

1985 The controversy surrounding the HIV/AIDS virus continues when Robert Gallo's lab patents an HIV test kit that later is approved by the FDA. The Pasteur Institute sues and is later awarded rights to half of the royalties from the new test. At the same time, HIV/AIDS enters the public eye when Rock Hudson dies of AIDS and Ryan White is barred from his elementary school in Indiana.

1987 A treatment arrives after 6 years of watching people die. This treatment is hailed as the first huge step in beating HIV/AIDS. The drug Retrovir (AZT, Zidovudine) is FDA approved and begins to be used in high doses to treat people infected with HIV. Politically, HIV/AIDS is a topic that most avoid. But in response to public pressure, President Ronald Reagan finally acknowledges the HIV/AIDS problem and for the

first time uses the term "AIDS" in a public speech. *100,000 to 150,000 cases of HIV and AIDS*
1990 After years of fighting to stay in school, and raging an even harder battle against the ravages of HIV/AIDS, Ryan White dies at the age of 19. That year, The Ryan White Care Act is enacted by Congress to provide government sponsored funds for the care of HIV/AIDS infected people *people living with HIV/AIDS rises to 1 million*
1992 The FDA approves the first drug to be used in combination with AZT. The addition of the drug Hivid marks the beginning of HIV/AIDS combination therapies. But a more disturbing development centers around HIV tainted blood. Three French senior health officials knowingly sell HIV tainted blood, resulting in the infection of hundreds of transfusion recipients, most of whom have hemophilia.
1993 Infected people and scientists alike are confused and concerned when a British study, the Concorde Trials, offers proof that AZT monotherapy does nothing to delay HIVS progression to AIDS in asymptomatic patients. As a result, the AZT debate emerges, with one side proclaiming AZT saves lives and the other denouncing AZT as useless; the "rethinker" movement is born.
1996 Treatment options take another step forward with the introduction of powerful HIV-fighting drugs called Protease Inhibitors. The use of these drugs in combination with existing HIV/AIDS drugs proves effective in controlling HIV. These new "triple-therapies" give patients and scientists new hope in eliminating HIV/AIDS. But that hope is dashed when, a year later, scientists find HIV/AIDS "hides" in reservoirs in the body, making total elimination of the virus virtually impossible.
1997 In late 1996, data from AIDS Clinical Trials Group study 076 (ACTG 076) made it clear that Retrovir (AZT) used during pregnancy and at the time of delivery drastically reduces transmission of HIV from mother to child. Those findings led to protocols that now drastically reduce transmission from mother to child from 1 in 4 to less than 3%.
1998 More than 15 years after the prediction that there would be an AIDS vaccine within two years, the first human trials in the United States of an HIV/AIDS vaccine begin. In a desperate attempt to get affordable HIV/AIDS drugs to the hardest hit areas of Africa, European drug companies ignore US patent laws and begin making generic versions of HIV/AIDS medications. In response, US drug companies file lawsuits to stop such practices. Sadly, 17 years after HIV/AIDS entered our culture, an African AIDS activist is beaten to death by neighbors after publicly admitting she was HIV infected.
2000 The AIDS "rethinker" movement gets international attention and support when

South African president Thabo Mbeki questions the use and effectiveness of HIV medications as well as offering doubt that HIV causes AIDS. In response, the international scientific community issues the Durban Declaration, offering proof that HIV and AIDS are indeed connected.

2001 As scientists become increasingly concerned about medication toxicity and effectiveness, US pharmaceutical companies drop their patent lawsuits, paving the way for European drug companies to manufacture and distribute cheaper HIV medications to the hardest hit areas of Sub-Saharan Africa. Cautious optimism emerges with the release of the first entry inhibitor, Fuzeon. Since 1981, 21 million people worldwide have died of AIDS, including 17 million from Sub-Saharan Africa. *31 million people are now living with HIV worldwide, the majority of whom are from African nations.*

2004 As the emphasis on simpler therapies continues, regimen pill burdens are greatly reduced with the release of two new combination drugs, Truvada and Epzicom and two new protease inhibitors, Revataz and Lexiva. The first generic formulation of an HIV medication is approved by the FDA, instilling hope that HIV medication prices may soon come down.

2005 HIV statistics have become sobering to say the least.
4.9 million people were newly infected in 2005.
40.3 million people worldwide living with HIV/AIDS.
As the numbers continue to climb, work on an HIV vaccine has for the most part failed. Once thought to be "just around the corner" it has become obvious that an HIV vaccine is still years away. Medication advances continue, but long-term side effects of HIV medication use are becoming more evident. So much so that experts now agree that for many patients, waiting to start HIV medications is the best course of action. Finally, 2005 saw a rise in HIV rates on college campuses, and risky behavior among those people already infected is still a problem. Positive prevention messages are becoming a priority as syphilis and other STD rates of infection continue to rise sharply.

2006 Experts conclude that HIV has its origins in the jungles of Africa among wild chimps. Experts go on to report that evidence suggests that the simian form of HIV (SIV) entered the human species and became HIV by way of monkey bites or ingesting monkey meat and brains. While the origins of HIV appear clearer, the means to pay for HIV care and medications have become more complicated. A revamping of the Medicare/Medicaid systems has made getting medications difficult for many. India surpasses South Africa as the world's largest HIV population, and, in

the US, infection rates of HIV are steady while STDs are on the rise.
2007 The Centers for Disease Control (CDC) reports that since the US HIV epidemic began, over 565,000 people have died of AIDS.
2009 Scientists at the University of North Carolina at Chapel Hill announce they have decoded the structure of an entire HIV genome. How this will affect the future of HIV treatment, prevention, and education is not entirely known. What is known is that the more professionals know about HIV, the better they can fight its effects on public health in the US and around the world.

Source: Cichocki, 2009

Advert (2011) reports the following events for years 2009 and fall 2010:

2009

- President Obama announces the removal of the travel ban that prevents HIV-positive people from entering the US.
- 4 million people in developing and transitional countries are receiving treatment for HIV; 9.5 million are still in immediate need of treatment.

2010

- The United States, South Korea, China and Namibia lift their travel bans for people living with HIV.
- The CAPRISA 004 microbicide trial is hailed a success after results show the gel reduced the risk of HIV infection by 40%.
- Results from the iPrEx trial show a reduction in HIV acquisition among men who have sex with men taking PrEP.

2011

- "The history of the domestic AIDS epidemic began in illness, fear, and
- death—but we conclude those 30 years with hope" (AIDS.GOV, 2011. pg. 1).

HIV/AIDS in Africa

The continent of Africa is known as the cradle of mankind. It is now widely, although controversially, accepted as the origin of HIV. This is an issue of great contention, especially with the stigma associated with HIV/AIDS. Opponents of the theory of the African origin of AIDS claim that this is part of the continued exploitation and stigmatization of both the continent and its people. Since Africa had survived slavery and colonialism, this school of thought adds, "The racist West deliberately and with malice aforethought, engineered and planted a lethal virus in Africa" (Muraah & Kiarie, 2001, pg. 6-7).

Avert (2009) reports that sub-Saharan Africa is more heavily affected by HIV and AIDS than any other region of the world. It is estimated that approximately two thirds of the total globe – that is around 22.4 million people are living with HIV in the region. In 2008, 1.9 people became infected and more than 14 million children have lost their parents. Since there are limited prevention and treatment services and programs, the numbers are expected to rise.

Sub-Saharan Africa faces triple challenges as identified below:

- Providing health care, antiretroviral treatment, and support to a growing population of people with HIV-related illnesses.
- Reducing the annual toll of new HIV infections by enabling individuals to protect themselves and others.
- Coping with the impact of over 20 million AIDS deaths, on orphans and other survivors, communities, and national development (Advert, 2009).

Impact of AIDS on Africa

Advert (2009) describes some of the major effects of the AIDS epidemic. Many parts of Africa are having widespread effects of the pandemic as identified below:

9

- The effect on life expectancy. In many countries of sub-Saharan Africa, AIDS is erasing decades of progress made in extending life expectancy. Millions of adults are dying from AIDS while they are still young or in early middle age. Average life expectancy in sub-Saharan Africa is now 47 years when it could have been 62 without AIDS.
- The effect on households. The effect of the AIDS epidemic on households can be very severe. Many families are losing their income earners. In other cases, people have to provide home-based care for sick relatives, reducing their capacity to earn money for their family. Many of those dying from AIDS have surviving partners, who are themselves infected and in need of care. They leave behind orphans, grieving and struggling to survive without a parent's care.
- The effect on healthcare. In all affected countries, the epidemic is putting a strain on the health sector. As the epidemic develops, the demand for care for those living with HIV rises, as does the number of health care workers affected.
- The effect on schools. Schools are heavily affected by AIDS. This a major concern because schools can play a vital role in reducing the impact of the epidemic through HIV education and support.
- The effect on productivity. The HIV and AIDS epidemic has dramatically affected labor, which in turn, slows down economic activity and social progress. The vast majority of people living with HIV and AIDS in Africa are between the ages of 15 and 49 – in the prime of their working lives. Employers, schools, factories, and hospitals have to train other staff to replace those at the workplace that become too ill to work.
- The effect on economic growth and development. The HIV and AIDS epidemic has already significantly affected Africa's economic development, and in turn, has affected Africa's ability to cope with the epidemic (Avert, 2009).

HIV/AIDS in Kenya

Kenya has a severe, generalized HIV epidemic. Ministry of Health (2005) reports a prevalence rate of eight percent in adult women and four percent in adult men. HIV/AIDS continues to be a challenge to Kenya's socioeconomic development. The first case was diagnosed in 1984, and it is now estimated that over 1.5 million people have died due to AIDS related illnesses and that 1.4 million people in Kenya are living with HIV today (National AIDS Control Council, 2005).

In March 2003, the current President of Kenya, Mwai Kibaki, declared "total war against HIV/AIDS" (PEPFAR, 2006, National AIDS Council, 2005). President Kibaki mandated the National AIDS Control Council to coordinate and manage the implementation of a multi-sectoral approach (including the development of strategic partnerships and mainstreaming HIV/AIDS in all key sectors) to HIV/AIDS to provide policy direction and mobilize resources (PEPFAR, 2006).

Since the first case was diagnosed in Kenya more than two decades ago, HIV/AIDS remains a problem for the country. In the beginning, many segments of the society expressed denial of the disease. Over time, the responses to the pandemic have evolved as many experienced sickness and death among family members. Kenya's political commitment was once limited; however, there are now numerous services that are in place to address the epidemic. There is still the issue of misconceptions, as many communities have not truly dealt with the disease (NASCOP, 2005). Unfortunately, women in Kenya face a higher risk of HIV infection than men, and they also experience a shorter life expectancy due to HIV/AIDS. According to the U. S. Department of State (2008), there is an HIV prevalence rate of eight percent in adult women and four percent in adult men. There are populations that are more at risk including injection drug users at fifty three percent and people in prostitution at twenty seven percent. In 2008 the Kenyan government sought to restructure many elements of the state. There were many constraints for controlling HIV/AIDS. The government determined the key to success would be developing effective training mechanisms for staff.

Women in Kenya and HIV/AIDS

Meaningful conversations about HIV and AIDS epidemic must incorporate an understanding of the role of women in Kenya (Heiser, 2010).

> I wish that you could come and be a part of seeing these women set free, not only from debt but from the enemy. Women over here are treated as chattel. A bride price is paid, and men that pay it "own" the women thereafter. It is a "normal" thing to beat your wife. In fact, if you don't, other men will condemn you and beat your wife for you. Men can have as many wives as they want, and if they don't legally marry the women, the women can be thrown out on the streets for as little as not cooking the way the husband likes. They have no recourse for support for themselves or the children born of these unions. Please pray for a change of heart in the men of this nation to see women the way God sees women, as precious gifts. I told a group the other day that so many young women, even as young as 10-12 years, are getting pregnant looking for love in all the wrong places. What does this say about the men here in Kenya? What does it say about the parents of these young women? Families sell their girls for as little as 100 shillings. That is about $1.10! They sell these young girls to old men, and some girls commit suicide instead of being imprisoned in such a relationship. In a primary school in one district, over a hundred young girls were impregnated by their teachers! It has become such a curse that the government is finally trying to take action against these predators. No longer are they going to let the predators pay a goat for them to be "forgiven" and not prosecuted (p. 1).

The National Council Women of Kenya (2006) suggests that women and girls are vulnerable to HIV/AIDS because of the "deep rooted gender inequalities in many Kenyan cultures." The Council identifies the following cultural practices and provides the following statistics:

- Female Genital Mutilation – 32% of women in Kenya are circumcised, and the average age of girls at the time of the procedure is between 7 -14 years old;
- 16% of currently married women in Kenya live in polygamous union;
- 20% of 15 – 19 year old girls in Kenya are currently or have been married. Often girls are married to older men, leaving them vulnerable to unequal power of their husbands; and
- Widow Inheritance – initiation of a new partner in relationship with a male partner; women have been forced to marry even when their husband dies of AIDS and they are infected.

Rape is also a problem in Kenya, although statistics are hard to obtain due to the culture of silence surrounding rape. According to the National Council Women of Kenya (2006), rape and HIV/AIDS are more complex than the risk of transmission as described below:

- In, 2003 there were 2308 cases of rape were reported to the authorities in Kenya;
- 25% of 12 -14 year olds lost their virginity by force;
- 4 out of t10 girls who have been raped suspect that they may have HIV/AIDS virus;
- A total of 3,097 cases of child defilement had been reported nation-wide between 2003 and 2004; and
- In Kenya 2/3 of women who are physically or sexually abused report their abusers to be their husbands or other relatives; 16% experience sexual violence.

The status and role of women in Kenya as caregivers is inextricably connected to their socio-economic status and cultural norms. Addressing HIV/AIDS must include an integrated dialogue that focuses on women.

Chapter 2

INSTITUTIONAL AND ORGANIZATIONAL RESPONSE TO HIV/AIDS

The entire community and its organizations and institutions are called upon to address the pandemic. Although community members have their unique roles, effective strategies require collective effort (Harambee). The following discussion provides specific discussion on the various partners in the effort to care for a community infected and affected by HIV and AIDS.

Role of the Church

Today, faith-based organizations play a leading role in the fight against HIV. You have an extensive network of people and institutions, especially in rural areas, where few other institutions exist. Many Africans are far more committed to their churches than to
    other social or political organizations. That is why so many churches and faith-based organizations have an incredible history of helping people with AIDS (UK International Development Secretary Hilary Benn, addressing the Church of England General Synod on HIV and AIDS, February 2004).
    A report, *Faith Untapped* (Tearfund, 2006) a faith-based nongovernmental organization indicated: "Churches have unparalleled influence and a long reach into remote areas ... for spreading messages about AIDS ... Crucially, churches are in a unique position to dispel the prejudice and gender inequality on which HIV and AIDS feed, provided they recognize the part they often play in reinforcing stigma and discrimination." According to the report, faith groups provide about 40 percent of healthcare in many African countries.

Spiritual/Pastoral Needs

Strengthening existing faith and helping People Living with HIV/AIDS (PLWHA) in spiritual growth boosts the spiritual aspect of life. This plays a great part in encouraging the person to have a positive view of life and to forgive others and self for any misconceptions and blames. The PLWHA will therefore be able to:

- Accept forgiveness by others.
- Forgive others.
- Have reassurance that God accepts them.
- Allow religious groups to offer support.
- Have freedom of worship according to faith, which should be respected by the health
- worker and the care providers.
- Call a religious leader of choice for sacraments counseling and other needs.

(Ministry of Health, 2002)

Churches in Kenya

In Kenya, there are more than 4000 churches (Churches in Kenya, 2010). In a study by Tearfund (2006), three key points were highlighted about the impact of HIV and AIDS in Africa as follows:

- Churches in Africa are a hidden and powerful force in tackling the HIV and AIDS crisis. They need international recognition, support and funding.
- Many churches contribute to the HIV and AIDS crisis through stigma and discrimination. Action is needed to overcome this.
- One of the single most effective areas into which churches could expand their HIV and AIDS work is preventing the virus from being passed from mothers to children.

Machyo (2001) asserts that the attitude of the Church should not be judgmental towards those living with AIDS, but should be based on witnessing God's unconditional love. The aforementioned author asserts that the Christian response to the AIDS pandemic is primarily about the extension of God's grace. The extension of grace can be established when churches start support groups that can reach out to people living with AIDS in their communities. The Church's great legacy from Jesus Christ is one of healing from all dimensions: "physical, psychological, social, environmental, moral, and spiritual" (page 1). Tearfund (2006) also addresses the need for supportive groups for those confronting the HIV/AIDS pandemic as suggested in the following statement:

> The churches and their vast networks of volunteers are one of the few groups which are wrestling with the pandemic at close quarters every single day. And yet they receive little recognition and scant funding from outside sources; in some cases churches' capacity is being stretched to breaking point. And yet churches are also part of the problem. Many people of faith need to think long and hard about the part they have played in feeding the stigma and discrimination surrounding HIV and AIDS. Churches represent vast untapped potential to change attitudes. If we put our own house in order and if we are properly resourced and trained, churches and other faith groups could become one of the single most effective strategies for tackling the pandemic (pg. 1).

There are the old denominations referred to as the mainstream churches in Kenya. The examples are:

- Roman Catholics
- Anglican Church
- Full Gospel Churches
- Presbyterian Church of East Africa
- Africa Inland Church
- Methodist

17

- Baptist

According to Churches in Kenya (2010), Kenya has witnessed an increase in the number of Pentecostal churches. Popular ones in Nairobi include:

- Nairobi Pentecostal Church
- Nairobi Lighthouse Church
- Redeemed Gospel Church
- Deliverance Church
- Jesus is Alive Ministries
- Jubilee Christian Centre

The Catholic Church

In December 1999, Catholic Bishops in Kenya wrote a pastoral letter acknowledging the challenge HIV/AIDS posed for the country. The letter called for recognition of the moral dimension of the disease and a collaborative effort between the Government, the youth, Christian communities, civic authorities, the media, health care workers, teachers, and educators in seeking solutions to the HIV/AIDS pandemic (Machyo, 2001). The Bishops used the following scripture to assert their responsibilities:

> … working together with all concerned, we hope to alleviate in all ways possible the moral, physical and spiritual suffering caused by the disease. We therefore exhort you in the words of our Lord Jesus Christ, Fear not, I am the first and the last; I am the living one! I was dead, but now I am alive forever and ever. I have authority over death and the world of the dead (Revelation. 1: 17-18)

The Catholic Church has taken the role of teacher regarding the HIV/AIDS pandemic. Catholic bishops and theologians have utilized the pandemic to reinforce traditional moral teachings and values. This is especially true regarding sexual behavior and marital relationships. The

Catholic Church has adopted some of the following strategies (Machyo, 2001)

- Prevention initiatives
- Provision of care for people living with HIV/AIDS
- Pastoral counseling
- Care for orphans

The Methodist Church

The overall aim of health programs established by the Methodist Church in Kenya (MCK) is to enable individuals and families to experience the fullness of life, which Christ came to bring (John 10:10) by promoting physical, mental, spiritual, and social health. The health activities of MCK are coordinated from the Conference Office by the Conference Health Coordinator and in collaboration with Conference Health Committees with representation from all the 10 Synods of the Church.

The Methodist Church has incorporated HIV/AIDS advocacy, support and care of the infected and affected persons in the society. These activities are coordinated by the HIV/AIDS Coordinator, who is currently based in Meru region (Methodist Church in Kenya, 2010). The Methodist Church has established the following health projects covering different parts of Kenya:

- Maua Methodist hospital and Palliative Care projects, Meru North
- Kenya Methodist University (KEMU) Health Program, Meru
- Mariene Methodist Clinic, Meru
- Laari HIV/AIDS program, Meru
- Kamwathu Clinic and Community projects, Tharaka
- Maburwa Community health project, Meru
- Kiandegwa Health Centre, Mwea, Embu
- Embu Mission Health Community Project, Eastern Kenya

- Kibera and Ngong Methodist Churches HIV/AIDS projects
- Itibo Dispensary, Kisii
- Igena Bamako Initiative, Kisii
- Shankoe Methodist Clinic, Transmara
- Enoretet Bamako Initiative, Transmara
- St. Paul Methodist Medical Clinic, Ugunja, Siaya
- Kilifi Orphan Project, Coast region
- Shirikisho Women Health project, Garsen, Lower Tana River
- HIV/AIDS Program in Primary Schools and Colleges in Kaaga and Mombasa

Through its Community Health Department, the hospital is actively involved in HIV/AIDS prevention, palliative, and home-based care projects as follows:

- Prevention of Mother to Child Transmission of HIV/AIDS in collaboration with Christian Health Association of Kenya was started at the same time with the Orphan project in 2001.
- Palliative care project in the hospital, churches and community.
- Community owned palliative care projects by the Churches in collaboration with Maua Hospital, which were started in 2002.
- Voluntary Counseling and Testing (VCTT) centers.
- Formation of support groups e.g. widows and widowers.

(Methodist Church in Kenya, 2010)

Faith Based Organization in Kenya

There are a numerous faith based organizations providing programs and services in Kenya. Examples of these organizations include:

- **Beacon of Hope** (BOH) "is a registered organization in Nairobi sharing the love of Christ in practical ways. The mission of BOH is to bring hope to women living with HIV/AIDS by equipping them to meet their spiritual, physical, emotional, and economic needs through: vocational training, product development and marketing, counseling, childcare, child education, and medical assistance" www.beaconafrica.org.

- **Life in Abundance International** (LIA) "exists to mobilize, train, and empower the indigenous/national-led church to improve the health and living standards of their neighbors through localized community development programs. Throughout the rural areas of Kenya, LIA facilitates community based orphan care and support" www.liaint.org.

- **Tanari Trust** "is a ministry of the Nairobi Baptist Church. The Trust provides camps, mentoring and discipleship for children orphaned by HIV/AIDS" www.tanari.org .

- **A Prepared Place** "facilitates adoptions of orphans for Christian families in Kenya. The organization also works to improve the infrastructure of the community in which it works by providing water and agricultural resources."

The Church must concentrate its efforts on educating and informing its people about prevention. It is necessary for information to be disseminated responsibly to avoid uncertainties and fears. Non-governmental AIDS organizations all over the world are beginning to conclude that prevention campaigns have not yielded the expected success based on the effort and money put into it. The meaning of knowledge may need to be redefined through accurate public awareness (Maluleke 2000).

There are dangerous traditional practices connected with the spread of the HIV/AIDS pandemic such as female circumcision, wife sharing and inheritance, sexual and economic subordination of women. The implications of these practices must be addressed. Baitu (2000) asserts that the

Catholic Church must go beyond emphasizing sexual abstinence before marriage and should emphasize African traditional structures such as the family and the community, which can advocate for the instruments of behavior that is imperative for decreasing the spread of HIV/AIDS.

A large percentage of monies that enable churches to continue to provide programs and services to address the HIV/AIDS pandemic comes from international donors. These donors should advocate on behalf of churches, stressing the unique contribution that churches are already making in response to HIV and AIDS in Africa. They should also recognize churches' potential to be even more effective with proper resourcing (Tearfund, 2006).

The Church and Family

God has uniquely prepared the Church to respond to this crisis and many parts of the Christian community in Africa. Oftentimes, the Church has responded with compassion, creativity, commitment, and courage. The following provides a synopsis of the impact the Church has had on the community:

- The church brings to the AIDS crisis a permanent presence at the grassroots level.
- The church has earned great respect in the community because of its compassion toward the weak and vulnerable in society, and, thus, has a powerful ability to influence on the individuals, the community and the nation.
- The church is an outstanding vehicle for getting information to the grassroots through its regular meetings.
- The church possesses an amazing ability to respond to crises through its abundant material resources and its army of compassionate volunteers (Pacanet, 2005).

The Church has also made a significant contribution to the HIV/AIDS pandemic as follows:

- The church has often been the first body to respond to the AIDS crisis.
- Individual Christians are leading many of the aspects of the HIV/AIDS battle across Africa.
- The Church, including its many denominations and NGO's, has led the way in taking care of orphans and vulnerable children.
- Compassionate Christians are the greatest single block of care givers for those affected by HIV/AIDS.
- The faith community and particularly the church is the best institution in society for encouraging behavioral change, which is often recognized as the single biggest need in preventing the spread of HIV (Pacanet, 2005).

If churches had the needed resources, they could have a profound impact on individuals and communities suffering from the HIV/AIDS pandemic. The three primary services needed would be prevention, care, and treatment as defined below:

- Prevention: churches have unparalleled influence and a long reach into remote areas. They have captive audiences and wide communication networks for spreading messages about AIDS.
- Care: church volunteers could move beyond offering counseling and moral support, to more proactive roles such as ensuring children in affected families can stay at school.
- Treatment: overstretched healthcare systems could delegate some testing and treatment services to community groups (Tearfund, 2006).

Mageto (2005) asserts that "A silent church = death" (p. 1). In the beginning of the epidemic, the church chose silence. The ministries of the Heiser's and Lynn Miller have recognized that the church must fight to overcome the spirit of silence as demonstrated through their ministries. Regardless of how uncomfortable it may be, churches must wake up from slumber and take their role in AIDS prevention and care. A large percentage of churches' belief has been that HIV/AIDS affects only the so-called risk groups, and there was a time that any attempt to respond to the crisis was seen as affirmation that a Western lifestyle is being practiced among the African people (Mageto, 2005).

Service Coordination and Implementation

Poor coordination of assistance provisions has negatively impacted HIV/AIDS service development and implementation. Kenya National HIV/AIDS Strategic Plan seeks to strengthen existing partnerships, networks, coordination mechanisms, and communication channels. Kenya's Minister of Health (2005) suggests that the time has come to harmonize interventions, asserting that it paramount that stakeholders at all levels work within a 'three-one' framework – one national coordinating body and authority, one national strategic plan, and one national monitoring and evaluation framework. However, there is often a lack of community involvement in contributing resources to support HIV/AIDS activities.

The National AIDS and STI Control Program (NASCOP) (2004) reports that a substantial number of effective Kenyan initiatives are in an unstable situation due to poor financing and wavering systems. Underlying difficulties contributing to financial problems include:

- Lack of systematic planning and budgeting
- Unreliable CBOs & NGOs funding systems
- Inadequate information regarding cost and effectiveness of program models
- Inconsistent approaches to providing services.

Limited staff and skills for management, support, and service delivery functions often remains a problem for program effectiveness. Ministry of Health services have limited staff numbers and skills at the health center level.

Retaining trained individuals is a significant challenge in communities and services NASCOP (2004).

An analysis was completed by NASCOP (2004) to identify gaps and difficulties regarding Home-based Care programs implementation and to determine where a number of systems are absent or undeveloped. Gaps identified included:

- Referral
- Networking, Coordination and Skill Transfer between Role Players
- NACC/Community Initiate Account Funding and Management
- Monitoring and Evaluation.

Non-Governmental Organizations in Kenya

In Kenya, a Non-Governmental Organization (NGO) is defined as a "private voluntary grouping of individuals or associations, not operated for profit or for other commercial purposes but which have organized themselves nationally or internationally for the promotion of social welfare, as well as development, charity, or research through mobilization of resources" (Haag, 2009, pg. 1). The World Bank (2011) asserts that the NGO consists of numerous types of organizations. NGOs range from large, Northern-based charities such as CARE, Oxfam and World Vision to community-based self-help groups in the South. They also include research institutes, churches, professional associations, and lobby groups. There are two main categories of NGOs: 1) **Operational** NGOs (primary purpose is the design and implementation of development-related projects), and 2) **advocacy** NGOs – (primary purpose is to defend or promote a specific cause and seek to influence policies and practices). Numerous NGOs engage in both operational and advocacy activities, and some advocacy groups. There are those who are not directly involved in the development and implementation of projects but focus on identified project-related concerns (World Bank, 2011).

NGOs have become increasingly involved in international development. Since the mid-1970s, there has been a substantial increase in the involvement of NGOs in developing countries. There was a -10 fold increase from 1970 to 1985 in developmental aid provided by international NGOs. In 1992 international NGOs contributed over $7.6 billion of aid to developing countries (World Bank, 2011). It is now estimated that more than 15 percent of total overseas development aid is channeled through NGOs. The aforementioned authors estimate that there are between 6,000 and 30,000 national NGOs in developing countries.

Operational NGOs

The World Bank categorized operational NGOs into three main groups as follows:

- **community-based** organizations (CBOs) - which serve a specific population in a narrow geographic area;
- **national** organizations - which operate in individual developing countries;
- **international** organizations - which are typically headquartered in developed countries and carry out operations in more than one developing country.

Throughout the 1970s and 1980s, most examples of World Bank-NGO collaboration involved international NGOs. However, in recent years there has been a reverse. There is an increase in the number of projects involved in community based organizations (World Bank, 2011).

Community Based Organizations (CBO) is also referred to as grassroots organizations or peoples' organizations. They usually require membership that is comprised of a group of individuals who have joined together to further their own interests CBOs are more likely to be the recipients of a project's goods and services. Many national and international NGOs work in partnership with CBOs through the distribution of resource, services and/or technical assistance (World Bank, 2011).

The following strength and weaknesses are associated with the NGO sector:

Strengths

- strong grassroots links and field-based development expertise
- the ability to innovate and adapt
- process-oriented approach to development
- participatory methodologies and tools
- long-term commitment and emphasis on sustainability
- cost-effectiveness

Weaknesses

- limited financial and management expertise
- limited institutional capacity
- low levels of self-sustainability
- isolation/lack of inter-organizational communication and/or coordination
- small scale interventions
- lack of understanding of the broader social or economic context

(World Bank, 2011).

In the last 20 years, NGOs have grown extensively in Kenya. There were 250 NGOs registered with the NGO Council of Kenya in 1993. In 10 years, the number multiplied to 2,323. Haag, (2009) suggests that this was mainly due to donor frustration in the early 1990s at government corruption, which resulted in the distributions of funds directly to NGOs in order to promote the New Policy Agenda of democratisation and good governance. This shift directly to NGO funding resulted in a substantial increase of

27

NGOs. Currently in Kenya, NGOs work across forty eight sectors including health accounting for 15% of all stated sectors; education 13%, environment 8.8%, relief/welfare 13%, and water 5.9%. Human Rights and minority groups including women's rights, children and disabled people account for 6.85% of all activity (Haag, 2009). Table 2 reflects NGOs in Kenya by sector.

Table 2:   NGO distribution by sector

NGO Activities	No of NGOs involved
Health	641
Education	645
AIDS	71
Welfare	445
Water and Sanitation	277
Human Rights	19
Women	129
Environment	414
Informal Sector	195
Relief	204
Social Services	212
Multi-sectoral	206
Population	110
Reproductive Health	20
Pastoralists/Arid Zones	105
Agriculture/Livestock	74
Food Security/Nutrition	24
Counseling/Mental Health	16
Enterprise	71
Income	16
Dev Ed	52

Religious	74
Youth/Child Rights	152
Culture and Arts	27
Disabilities	22
Research	51
Legal	12
Peace and Conflict	15
Housing	5
Land Rights	1
Energy	2
Fisheries	2
Drugs	6
Family	34
Leadership	3
Wildlife	13
Nature Conservation	27
Forestry	17
Media and Communications	19
Appropriate Technology	10
Information Technology	51
Consumer	8
Transport	12
Sports and Leisure	14
Social Policy	6
Refugees	48
Emergency	13
Vets	2
Rural Development	215

Source: Haag, 2009

Many of the NGOs have offices in Nairobi. As reflected in Table 2, they often conduct high-impact, high-resource projects and operate in the fields of health, refugees, environment, human rights, education, and other key aspects of international development (Haag, 2010). Social workers play a vital role in addressing issues related to international development through the implementation of programs/services and serving as a voice of advocacy.

International Social Work

The establishment of social work programs worldwide has grown astronomically in the last 20 years. The North Carolina Chapter of the National Association of Social Work (NASW, 2010) reports that Social Workers have heeded the call regarding the need for implementation of programs and policies focusing on disenfranchised groups globally. International social work goes beyond the needs of the people in the United States and looks at people around the world that need help. International social work looks at the immediate emergencies that happen around the world and everyday problems that people in other countries have to live within their everyday lives. International social work promotes social changes where they are necessary, helps to solve problems in human relationships, and to enhance the wellbeing of people's lives.

The Council on Social Work Education (CSWE) has commissioned social workers to meet the global needs of disenfranchised groups in societies. The recent accreditation standards have incorporated a global component (CSWE, 2010).

International Institute

In 2004, the CSWE established The Katherine A. Kendall Institute for International Social Work Education with an endowment from the Katherine A. Kendall Fund. The overall mission is to integrate international content in social work education and to increase the cross-organizational collaboration in project development, as well as research and data collection and dissemination. Specifically, it promotes the implementation of programs and initiatives within the global social work education community. These programs and initiatives will prepare practitioners and researchers with the appropriate knowledge and requisite skills for practice within an increasingly interdependent global community.

Institute Goals

Promote standards of excellence for international work
Conduct faculty development initiatives for internationalizing the curriculum
Foster greater connections between CSWE and other international social work organizations, such as the International Association of Schools of Social Work (IASSW)
Maintain a database of curriculum resources and international initiatives that are taking place in U.S. social work programs
Publish educational materials for internationalizing the curriculum
Plan annual seminars with invited experts in global economics and social development in order to enrich perspectives and understandings

(CSWE, 2010)
Commission on Global Education

The Commission on Global Social Work Education works with other international organizations, including the International Association of Schools of Social Work (IASSW) to promote international programs and projects and to develop the international dimension of the social work curricula. The commission is also responsible for advising the Foreign Equivalency Determination Service and maintaining relationships with foreign students and schools (Commission on Global Education, 2010).

Council on Global Learning, Research and Practice

The Council on Global Learning, Research, and Practice is one of the councils of the Commission on Global Social Work Education. The following are the specific charges of the Council:

- Collaborate with the Commission on Professional Development to initiate and facilitate faculty development programs in global social work
- Promote development of social workers competent in international practice
- Develop a database of existing international activity in member programs to function as a resource for further development
- Identity key global issues and events and their impact on social work education. Publish educational materials for globalizing the curriculum
- Plan seminars
- Provide leadership in universalizing the global perspective in the social work curriculum
- Promote standards of excellence of international social work
- Develop resources and guidelines for International Field Placements
- Work to guarantee the infusion of global social work throughout CSWE

(CSWE, 2010).

International Association of Schools of Social Work

The mission of the International Association of Social Workers (IASSW) is to promote a worldwide excellence in social work education and engagement of a community of social work educators in international exchange of information and expertise.

IASSW carries out its purposes through:

- a biennial conference of social work educators, the IASSW Congress
- publication of a newsletter
- representation at the United Nations
- co-sponsorship with IFSW and ICSW of the journal International Social Work
- activities of Committees and Task Forces
- funding of small cross-national projects in social work education

Important recent policy documents include the Definition of Social Work, Global Standards for Social Work Education and Training, and Ethics in Social Work: Statement of Principles (all developed with the International Federation of Social Workers).

IASSW was founded in 1928 at the First International Conference of Social Work, which was held in Paris. It was initially comprised of 51 schools, mostly in Europe, and was known as the International Committee. Revitalized after World War II, the organization expanded its membership to include a wider range of countries and was renamed the International Association of Schools of Social Work. The association has member schools in all parts of the world, including five regional organizations in Africa, Asia and the Pacific, Europe, Latin America, and North America and the Caribbean. These associations are affiliated with the IASSW and represented on the Board of Directors (International Association of Schools of Social Work, 2010).

International Federation of Social Workers

The International Federation of Social Workers (IFSW) is a global organization, which strives for social justice, human rights, and social development through the development of social work best practices and international cooperation between social workers and their professional organizations. IFSW is a successor to the International Permanent Secretariat of Social Workers, which was founded in Paris in

1928 and was active until the outbreak of World War II. It was not until 1950, at the time of the International Conference of Social Work in Paris, that the decision was made to create the IFSW. All over the world, people are being harmed, abused, and neglected and their civil, political, economic, cultural, and social rights are being violated (IFSW, 2010).

Chapter 3

HIV/AIDS PATIENTS AND THEIR CAREGIVERS

"Neither words nor statistics can adequately capture the human tragedy of children grieving for dying or dead parents, stigmatized by society through association with AIDS, plunged into economic crisis and insecurity by their parent's death and struggling without services or support systems in impoverished communities" (Muchiri, 2002 p. 2).

Fear and ignorance have severe effects on the individual, family, group and, society levels. HIV/AIDS patients are often neglected in their families and communities; however, they require extensive support and care through HIV/AIDS programs to address this "pandemic." Some programs deal with prevention and control through awareness campaigns and counseling services. Others are home-based care programs, which allow HIV/AIDS patients to be taken care of in their own homes. In all of these great efforts, the "caregiver" has no support system and is neglected at the expense of the magnitude of the effects of HIV/AIDS (Muchiri, 2002).

True response to the breaking of silence of the HIV/AIDS pandemic requires an integrated approach to the whole question of HIV/AIDS. While it is imperative to provide care to the HIV patient, it is essential that there is also a focus on the needs of caregivers. Caregivers are an integral part in the fight against HIV/AIDS (Muchiri, 2002). Caregivers often become their own worst enemy, holding themselves to impossible standards (Check, 1989). Tenseness, anger, frustration, guilt, and sadness are normal responses to the strain of living with and caring for an HIV/AIDS patient. The constant demands of care giving can and does lead to emotional and physical fatigue, especially when providing care for individuals suffering from terminal illnesses. Cohen & Eisdoxer (1986) suggests that the way to deal with the difficulties of caregiving successfully is to recognize that the caregiver role is impossible to fulfill in its entirety, but one must try to do the best that he/she can.

Caregivers face many risks in communities of Kenya. Cultural beliefs and practices detrimental to good caregiving practices should be discouraged. Onyango's (2008) findings from fourteen HIV+ caregivers' research participants claimed that their infections were due to caregiving for PLWHA. The development and implementation of home-based care programs is important for both patients and families. They are an essential component of reducing risks to the caregivers.

Home-Based Care and Caregivers

In order for home-based caregivers to be effective, they must have adequate resources and training. There is also a need for improved continuity of care. Systems must be able to effectively work together (i.e. the hospitals, community facilities, and the home). In Kenya, community participation in caregiving for PLWHA's is often limited. This leaves the caregiving responsibility to the immediate family members, often very young children and old women (Onyango, 2008; HGO Focus Groups, 2006).

While home-based care provides a number of benefits to the HIV/AIDS patients, further investigation must take place regarding the effects of the role on caregivers. There are potential risks to home-based caregivers. Without inter-ventions that stress health education, health promotions, and training on the best practices of caregiving, caregivers are at risk of suffering from ailments and infection. Supervision of caregivers is needed to increase their knowledge and skills. There is also a great need for advocacy by policy makers to improve the working conditions of home-based caregivers. Often families of PLWHAs do not have access to food, water, and sanitation to reduce caregiver's responsibilities (Onyango, 2008; HGO Focus Groups, 2006). Numerous factors have led to the promotion of HIV/-AIDS' home-based care programs. Inability of both patients and relatives to pay hospital bills and an overstretched health care system have provided for alternative methods of HIV patients' care (Muraah & Kiarie, 2001). Home-based care provides patients with support from family and friends that a hospital cannot offer. Home-based care programs provide HIV/AIDS patients with a sense of belonging and significantly reduce travel expenses to and from the hospital for the patients and their caregivers (Muraah & Kiare, 2001).

Training and involvement of caregivers and volunteers can significantly reduce the cost of sustaining community based care programs (National AIDS and STI Control Program, 2004 and Muraah & Kiarie, 2001). A community can provide caregivers with positive encouragement that may reduce the HIV related stigma and encourage changes in traditional practices that increase risk of HIV infection. It has been established that the affected family's greatest worry is not just the HIV infection but also the impact the disease has on their income.

What Is Home-Based Care?

Home-based care is an approach to care provision that combines clinical services, nursing care, counseling, and social support. It represents a continuum of care from the health facility, to the community to the family, to the individual infected with HIV/AIDS, and back again. The Kenyan government is committed to home-based care as a viable mechanism for delivering services because it has important benefits for everyone on that continuum (Ministry of Health, 2002).

Home-based long-term care is the care necessary for people of all ages, who have chronic health problems and need assistance with activities of daily living (ADLs) in order to enjoy a reasonable quality of life (WHO, 2000; Kenya Ministry of Health, 2002). Home-based health care encourages the comfort of familiar environments, keeps the patient's family and social relationships intact, and is, therefore, most often the preferred alternative to institutional care. However, the type and duration of illness can put specific demands on families (WHO, 1999). In order to truly be effective, home-based care must be extended from the health facility to the patients' home through family participation and community involvement within available resources and in collaboration with health care workers.

Kenya Ministry of Health (2002) encourages home-based care that is a holistic, collaborative effort by the hospital, the family of the patient, and incorporates the community to enhance the quality of life of PLWHAs and their families. Comprehensive care is across the continuum of care from the health facility through to community/home level. It encompasses clinical care, nursing care, counseling and psycho-spiritual care, and social support. The emphasis of each is as follows:

Clinical care: Includes early diagnosis, rational treatment, and planning for follow-up care of HIV-related illness.
Nursing care: Includes care to promote and maintain good health, hygiene, and nutrition.
Counseling and psycho-spiritual care: Includes reducing stress and anxiety for both PLWHAs and families, promoting positive living, and helping individuals to make informed decisions on HIV testing, planning for the future and behavioral changes, making risk reduction plans, and involving sexual partner(s) in such decisions.
Social support: Includes information and referral to support groups, welfare services, and legal advice for individuals and families, including surviving family members, and, where feasible, provision of material assistance.

(Ministry of Health, 2002)

Objectives of Home-Based Care

The primary identified focus of Home-Based Care services in Kenya includes the following:

- To facilitate the continuity of the patients care from the health facility to the home and community.
- To promote family and community awareness of HIV/AIDS prevention and care.

- To empower the PLWHA, the family, and the community with the knowledge needed to ensure long-term care and support.
- To raise the acceptability of PLWHAs by the family/community, hence reducing the stigma associated with AIDS.
- To streamline the patient/client referral from the institutions into the community and from the community to appropriate health and social facilities.
- To facilitate quality community care for the infected and affected.
- To mobilize the resources necessary for sustainability of the service.

Principles of Home-Based Care

To ensure that the foregoing benefits are realized, home-based care must be regarded as a holistic system of care with provisions for the following:

- Ensuring appropriate, cost-effective access to quality health care and support to enable persons living with HIV/AIDS to retain their self-sufficiency and maintain quality of life.
- Encouraging the active participation and involvement of those most affected (those
- living with HIV/AIDS).

- Fostering the active participation and involvement of those most able to provide
- support to the community at all levels.
- Targeting social assistance to all affected families, especially children.
- Caring for caregivers, in order to minimize the physical and spiritual exhaustion that can come with the prolonged care of the terminally ill.
- Ensuring respect for the basic human rights of PLWHAs.
- Developing the vital role of home-based care as the link between prevention and care.
- Taking a multi-sector approach to care and support.
- Addressing the reproductive health and family planning needs of persons living with HIV/AIDS.
- Instituting measures to ensure the economic sustainability of home care support.
- Building and supporting referral networks/linkages and collaboration among participating entities.
- Building capacity at all levels – household, community, institution.
- Addressing the differential gender impact of the HIV/AIDS epidemic and care for persons living with HIV/AIDS.

(Ministry of Health, 2002)

The HIV/AIDS pandemic in Kenya has required the development and implementation of home-based care as an alternative way of managing infected patients. These individuals often remain ill for prolonged durations. The burden on health facilities is high; more than 50% of bed-occupancy in most government hospitals is from patients suffering from HIV/AIDS-related infections. These patients occupy beds for long periods and on repeated occasions, due to the frequent re-occurrence of the opportunistic diseases that inflict them (Crouch, 2002). The patients require extended periods of health care, along with emotional and social support, and the busy, overworked hospital staff may not be able to provide this.

In 2002, Kenya's Ministry of Health introduced a home-based health care initiative in an effort to reduce bed-occupancy in government health facilities. The rationale behind the efforts was that home was a supportive and caring environment. Consequently, many AIDS-Related Infections (ARI) patients, most of whom were women, were discharged to home to be nursed by their relatives (Ministry of Health, 2003). While patients feel comfortable among their family at home, there is often a lack of the basic resources essential for long-term home-based care. Due to poverty, there is not adequate nutritious food, clean drinking water and sanitation, and protective clothing like hand gloves for use when handling these patients (HGO Focus Groups, 2006). Murah & Kiarie (2001) assert that *successful* home-based care programs must:

- Make sure that patients get adequate nursing and other support necessary to cope with the disease;
- Make it possible for healthcare personnel to make house calls;
- Train volunteers, HIV patients and close relatives in basic patient care and infection control;
- Combine care with HIV prevention initiatives;
- Encourage acceptance of HIV/AIDS patients by the community
- Reduce overcrowding in hospitals, thus freeing resources for the management of other diseases;
- Promote good nutrition and personal hygiene; and
- Encourage and motivate the HIV patients (p. 110)

Utilization of basic medical supplies and nursing skills can give caregivers the means to provide quality home-based care to HIV patients.

How to Organize Home-Based Care?

Strategic partnerships among family members, health care workers, local communities, community-based organizations (CBOs), non-government organizations (NGOs), and those living with HIV/AIDS in providing care and support to those infected and affected by the HIV/AIDS epidemic are imperative for the success of home-based care programs. Effective community home-based care programs must incorporate two strengths that exist throughout the world: families and communities. Families are the central focus of care and should form the basics of the family/community health based team (African Council of Aids Service Organizations, 2009).

Communities often provide a source of support and care to individuals and families in need. The primary goal of community home-based care programs are to offer hope through quality and suitable care. This will enable family caregivers and their sick family members to maintain independence and achieve the best possible quality of life. Also, their loved ones will be able to maintain their dignity.

Care that is embraced by the community encourages the reduction of stigma and discrimination against PLWHA. The further spread of the virus is often reduced as well as the negative the impact of HIV/AIDS on individuals, families, and communities. With the promotion of community participation, family and community members are empowered. The relative has the option of caring for the PLWHA at convenient times, while also accommodating other household commitments. When there is effective coordination with health facilities through an effective referral system, community home-based programs complement formal health structures (African Council of AIDS Service Organizations, 2009).

Home-based care needs can be identified as those specific to the PLWHA, to the family, and to the community within which the PLWHA lives. These needs may be physical, spiritual/pastoral, social, or psychological but will vary from person to person and from one community to the other. These needs should be identified when a PLWHA is being enrolled into a home-based care program, for example while still in hospital, in an effort to ensure proper planning and integration of activities. Early identification also ensures adequate resource mobilization and the sustainability of activities initiated.

Presidents Emergency Plan for AIDS Relief

In 2003, the U.S. President's Emergency Plan for AIDS Relief (PEPFAR) was launched to combat global HIV/AIDS – the largest commitment by any nation to combat a single disease in history. Congress's findings provided justification as indicated in the table below:

Table 3:   PEPFAR

(1) During the last 20 years, HIV/AIDS has assumed pandemic proportions, spreading from the most severely affected regions, sub-Saharan Africa and the Caribbean, to all corners of the world, and leaving an unprecedented path of death and devastation.
(2) According to the Joint United Nations Program on HIV/AIDS (UNAIDS), more than 65,000,000 individuals worldwide have been infected with HIV since the epidemic began, more than 25,000,000 of these individuals have lost their lives to the disease, and more than 14,000,000 children have been orphaned by the disease. HIV/AIDS is the fourth-highest cause of death in the world.
(3)(A) At the end of 2002, an estimated 42,000,000 individuals were infected with HIV or living with AIDS, of which more than 75 percent live in Africa or the Caribbean. Of these individuals, more than 3,200,000 were children under the age of 15 and more than 19,200,000 were women.
(3)(B) Women are four times more vulnerable to infection than men and are becoming infected at increasingly high rates, in part because many societies do not provide poor women and young girls with the social, legal, and cultural protections against high risk activities that expose them to HIV/AIDS.
(3)(C) Women and children who are refugees or are internally displaced persons are especially vulnerable to sexual exploitation and violence, thereby increasing the

43

possibility of HIV infection.
(4) As the leading cause of death in sub-Saharan Africa, AIDS has killed more than 19,400,000 individuals (more than 3 times the number of AIDS deaths in the rest of the world) and will claim the lives of one-quarter of the population, mostly adults, in the next decade.
(5) An estimated 2,000,000 individuals in Latin America and the Caribbean and another 7,100,000 individuals in Asia and the Pacific region are infected with HIV or living with AIDS. Infection rates are rising alarmingly in Eastern Europe (especially in the Russian Federation), Central Asia, and China.
(6) HIV/AIDS threatens personal security by affecting the health, lifespan, and productive capacity of the individual and the social cohesion and economic well-being of the family.
(7) HIV/AIDS undermines the economic security of a country and individual businesses in that country by weakening the productivity and longevity of the labor force across a broad array of economic sectors and by reducing the potential for economic growth over the long term.
(8) HIV/AIDS destabilizes communities by striking at the most mobile and educated members of society, many of whom are responsible for security at the local level and governance.

Source: PEPFAR, 2010

PEPFAR/PFWHA

Palliative care under PEPFAR is "a comprehensive approach to providing services, which support quality of life for HIV-positive adults and children" (PEPFAR, 2009 pg. 1). Traditional palliative care usually focuses on pain and symptom relief at the end of life. PEPFAR programs have a holistic view, incorporating clinical, psychological, spiritual, social and preventive care services (PEPFAR, 2009). The figure below is the *Continuum of Care – Optimal* model for the palliative care program adapted from Frank D. Ferris (2000). The model blends curative practices with comfort care, i.e. palliative care.

Figure 2:   Continuum of Care

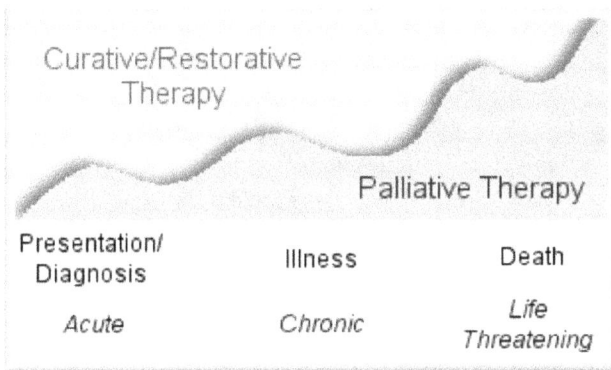

Figure 2. Adapted from Frank D. Ferris, 2000.

Comfort care related to HIV/AIDS begins when there is an HIV positive diagnosis. The care then extends to the death of the individual. With comfort care practice, there is a focus on family centered approaches. PEPFAR has identified the following as palliative care activities:

- Clinical services include preventive care with antibiotic prophylaxis for opportunistic infections (i.e. cotrimoxazole), insecticide-treated nets, and interventions to improve the quality of drinking water and hygienic practices; treatment and care services for opportunistic infections; pain alleviation and symptom management nutritional counseling assessment and rehabilitation for malnourishment; routine clinical monitoring, including evaluating the need for ART; support for ART adherence; and end-of-life care. PEPFAR supports work with policy makers to develop appropriate policies related to antibiotic prophylaxis and pain control.

- Social care supports community mobilization, leadership development for people living with HIV/AIDS, legal services, linkages to food support and income-generating programs, and other activities to strengthen households and communities.

- Psychological services provide mental health counseling, family care and support groups, memory books, cultural and age-specific approaches for psychological care, identification and treatment of HIV-related psychiatric illnesses, and bereavement preparedness.
- Spiritual care includes assessment, counseling, facilitating forgiveness, and life completion tasks.
- Positive prevention efforts should be incorporated across the spectrum of palliative care services to reduce the risk of transmitting HIV from HIV-positive persons to others. These services include counseling and HIV testing for the entire family, prevention counseling and services, and biomedical interventions that reduce transmission risk (i.e. treatment of sexually transmitted diseases) (PEPFAR, 2009).

In 2004, Kenya received nearly $92.5 million under PEPFAR; in Fiscal Year (FY) 2004, more than $142.9 million; in FY2005, approximately $208.3 million; in FY2006, and $368.1 million in FY2007 to support comprehensive HIV/AIDS prevention, treatment, and care programs. PEPFAR provided nearly $534.8 million in FY2008. Also, as of September 30, 2008, PEPFAR has supported care for more than 10.1 million people affected by HIV/AIDS worldwide. This number includes more than 4 million orphans and vulnerable children. Through September 30, 2008, PEPFAR supported training or retraining of 462,500 individuals to care for people living with HIV/AIDS.

PEPFAR Progress Achieved in Kenya:

- 229,700 individuals receiving antiretroviral treatment as of September 30, 2008
- 540,300 HIV-positive individuals received care and support in FY2008 (including TB/HIV)
- 533,700 orphans and vulnerable children (OVCs) were served by an OVC program in FY2008

- 3,000,800 pregnant women receiving HIV counseling and testing services for prevention of mother-to-child HIV transmission (PMTCT) since the beginning of PEPFAR
- 182,700 HIV-positive pregnant women receiving antiretroviral prophylaxis for PMTCT since the beginning of PEPFAR
- 1,722,400 counseling and testing encounters (in settings other than PMTCT) in FY2008
- 4,574,300 individuals reached with community outreach HIV/AIDS prevention programs that promote Abstinence and/or Being Faithful in FY2008
- 5,941,000 individuals reached with community outreach HIV/AIDS prevention activities that promote Condoms and related prevention services in FY2008
- 40,002,000 USG condoms shipped from Calendar Year 2004 to 2008

These successes document both progress and gaps in services and resources needed to conquer the pandemic.

Chapter 4

OVERVIEW OF CAREGIVERS' STUDY

The Kenya National AIDS Control Council (NACC) requested "the development of innovative responses to reduce the impact of the epidemic on communities, social services, and economic productivity," targeting vulnerable groups including caregivers (NACC, 2005, pg. 29). In response to the call of the NACC and the funding opportunities for services provided by PEPFAR, Higher Ground Outreach, Inc. responded to the appeal by reaching out to partner with Faith and Community Based Organizations in Kenya to provide services to HIV/AIDS patients and their caregivers. Building upon this commitment, HGO commissioned a series of HIV/AIDS caregiver focus groups to gain a better understanding of the challenges associated with HIV/AIDS caregiving and to develop a plan of action to implement appropriate programs and services.

Participant Selection

Country Side Widows and Orphans Enterprises (COSWE), an organization registered under Kenya's Non-Governmental Organizations Bureau (NGO) served as the host for this research. The following steps were utilized by COSWE and HGO for this exploratory study:

- Contacted the Ministry of Social Services/Com–missioner for Social Services who encouraged COSWE to get a permit for the research.
- Applied for permit from the Ministry of Education and was given permit to carry out the research for 6 weeks.
- Ministry of Education provided COSWE/HGO with a letter of introduction to be presented to the Department of

Education and Department of Public Health in Nairobi, Provincial Administration Office.

*   Approached programs that are hosting HIV/AIDS programs in Nairobi, specifically approaching a variety of Faith Based Organizations (FBO) and NGOs to recruit HIV/AIDS Caregivers to participate in the Focus Group Discussion
*   Appointed a representative from each identified agency that was willing to recruit HIV/AIDS Caregivers to participate in the program.
*   COSWE coordinated two separate discussion forums with FBOs and NGOs – the organizations were selected based on HIV/AIDS services provided in the community.

Description of FBO and NGOs Participating in the Study

The following is a brief description of the Faith Based and Non-governmental organizations participating in the research with additional information described in Table 4.

The Kariobangi HIV/AIDS Program:

Kariobangi HIV/AIDS Program is located in Kariobangi. The area is a low-income residential estate in northeastern Nairobi, Kenya. It comprises both apartments and slum-type dwellings (Maps of the World, 2011). The program is sponsored by the Friends Community Congregation. Participants for the focus group were recruited by the program's coordinator.

WEMA Center:

The WEMA Center is located in the Thika District. There are pockets of extreme poverty found mainly in the urban slums in Thika Municipality, Ruiru Town, and Juja. Some 48.4% of the population in the whole district is under absolute poverty and poverty incidence is on the increase, due to factors such as unemployment, collapse of agricultural sector, collapse of industries, poor infrastructure, and the rise in HIV/AIDS (WEMA Centre, 2011). Participants for the focus group were recruited by the project coordinator.

Champions of Christ

Champions of Christ is located in Athi River Division. It is a part of the Machakos County. The most prevalent diseases are Malaria and skin diseases. HIV/AIDs in Machakos is a major health problem with the prevalence rate averaging 15%. Approximately 50% of the hospital beds are occupied by patients with HIV/AIDs- related diseases. HIV\AIDS in the county was first diagnosed in June 1989, at which time 4 males and 5 females tested HIV positive (Softkenya.com, 2011). Participants for the focus group were recruited by the project coordinator.

St. Michael Catholic Church

St. Michael Catholic Church HIV/AIDS Support Program is located in Kibera. Kibera is a densely populated slum that is socially and economically vulnerable. Residents live in extremely precarious conditions where health, sanitation, and infrastructure are non-existent. Disease is rife, with the biggest killer in the slum being HIV/AIDS-related diseases (Med.Net, 2004). The focus group participants were recruited by the project's full-time nurse.

Table 4 describes the agencies that were utilized to recruit HIV/AIDS caregivers and their recruitment strategies.

Protocol

Through phone calls and organization letters, COSWE confirmed the planned attendance from each recruited organization. The moderators explained the purpose of the Focus Group and reviewed the research consent form both in Swahili and English. By their signature on the sign-in sheet, participants agreed to participate and abide by the rules of confidentiality; participants were informed that they would receive 100 shillings to purchase lunch. The sessions were audio recorded.

Table 4: NGO Caregiver Recruitment

NGOs & FBOs	Description of Agency	HIV/AIDS Caregiver Recruitment Strategy
KARIOBANGI HIV/AIDS Program	Program supported by the Friends Church Congregation for low income communities. The program currently provides care to 700 orphans. Approximately 350 of the orphans are HIV/AIDS patients.	The Organization's Project Coordinator recruited HIV/AIDS caregivers from individuals participating in the program.
WEMA Center	An HIV/AIDS program Supported by the Nairobi Community. WEMA provides support to 382 orphans whose parents have died from AIDS. Approximately 20% of the orphans are infected with HIV.	The Organization's Project Coordinator recruited HIV/AIDS caregivers from individuals participating in the program.
Champions of Christ	An HIV/AIDS project for support to families of HIV/AIDS patients located in the Athi River Division, which includes 10 slums. HIV/AIDS contributes to 30% of the orphans in the community.	The Organization's Project Coordinator recruited HIV/AIDS caregivers from individuals participating in their Caregiver Support Group.
St. Michael's Catholic Church HIV/AIDS Support Program	Initiative for empowering HIV/AIDS patients with origins from the Kibera Slums, Kibera is the largest 'slum' area in East and Central Africa.	The Priest appointed the project's full-time nurse to recruit HIV/AIDS caregivers residing in the Kibera Community.

Source: HGO Focus Groups, 2006

The facilitators utilized a Moderator's Guide, which included six discussion questions (with prompts) developed by Dr. Sandra Edmonds Crewe, Professor, Howard University School of Social Work. The guide was originally used in a 2003 AARP Grandparent Caregiver study and included seven questions; however, only six were utilized in this study. Input on the six discussion questions was provided by the Kenya Commissioner of Social Services and two Master Level Kenyan Social Workers with extensive experience working HIV/AIDS patients and teaching at various universities in Kenya. Based on their feedback, the guide was slightly modified to reflect cultural sensitivity.

Crewe (2003:6) asserts that "Rituals such as greeting participants and acknowledging their (focus group participants') values are critically important in getting them to be open and honest with the process." It is imperative that a sense of trust is established by the moderators. Cultural sensitivity is also essential; the fact that one of the Moderators was a Kenyan Social Worker enabled the participants to be more receptive and have a sense of comfort.

Research Limitations

The research could have been strengthened by administering a survey that measured caregiver burden. The qualitative comments provide rich information; however, using an instrument to measure burden would have been helpful with the analysis. Additional depression or other mental health scales could have been used to better explore previous findings that informal caregivers of HIV patients may benefit from mental health services because of the depressive symptoms (Pirraglia, Bishop, Herman, Trisvan, Lopez, Torgersen 2005).

Additionally, the study included important information on both female and male caregivers. Because the data was grouped with no differentiation between comments from males and females, no findings could be isolated that addressed gender-roles. Other research on caregiving and AIDS patients in Uganda has suggested that "making the involvement of men in the care of sick family members more culturally acceptable could substantially alleviate some of the women's heavy work load and free their time for other essential family health tasks such as caring for young children" (Kipp, Tindyebam, Karamagi, & Ruballe, 2006, p. 3). The absence of this detail prevented this analysis.

Finally, the research could have been strengthened by connecting the findings with the specific groups attached to the focus groups. There was some evidence that FBOS and NGOs may have served caregivers with different perspectives about their roles; however, the transcripts did not identify the caregivers by group.

HIV/AIDS Caregiver Identified Demographic Information

There were four caregiver focus groups and participants, who ranged in age from 16 to 80 years. Almost 80% were females and just over 20% were males. The 116 care receivers were relatives (41.3%), friends (40.5%), and neighbors (18.1%). They ranged in age from 1 to 55 years of age. It is important to note that the majority of care receivers (81.8%) were identified as friends and neighbors and not relatives. Also, approximately one-third (32.5%) indicated that they were employed, 53.6% indicated that they were unemployed, and 16.2% indicated that they were volunteers. It cannot be determined whether they were employed or not. However, 41.8% of the caregivers reported no income. More than 30% of the caregivers were married, 16% were widowed, 12% separated or divorced, and 42% were single. Two of the focus groups had teen caregivers. Table 5 and Figure1 reflect the HIV/AIDS Caregiver Participants' demographic information.

The additional demographic data below provides context about the circumstances of caregivers in the study. Most have children and have between 12 and 16 members in their households. Also, they report caregiving between 3 and 15 years.

Figure 3: Focus Group Demographic Information

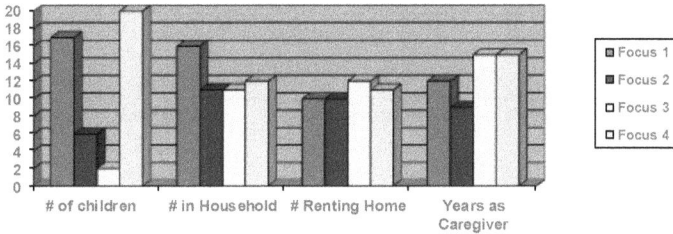

The focus group participants, like the caregivers in Kenya, are mostly women. The majority of the care for people living with HIV takes place in the home, and up to 90% of that is provided by women and girls in the countries hardest hit. Older women are providing care on an unprecedented scale, assuming responsibility not only for their children and grandchildren, but also for other children orphaned and made vulnerable by AIDS. There are more working age women living with HIV. They constantly struggle to provide for their families, but they are often in need of care themselves. As a result, caregiving duties shift increasingly to older women and younger girls. This makes HIV and AIDS a gender justice concern given the other inequities in the communities (UN AIDS, 2006).

Table 5: HIV/AIDS Caregiver Demographic Information

Focus Groups	Caregiver Participants	Relationship to Patient	Income Per Month (Shillings)	Employment Status	Marital Status
Focus Group 1 Kario-bangi N= 10	7 Female 3 Male Ages 16-62	11 Relatives 1 Neighbor 1 Friend Ages Indicated 1-47	4 None 2 100 1 2000 2 3000 1 N/A	5 Employed 5 Unem-ployed	4 Married 1 Widow 5 Single
Focus Group 2 WEMA N= 10	8 Female 2 Male Ages 16-62	2 Relatives 8 Neighbors 21 Friends Ages Indicated 6-55	5 None 1 1000 2 1200 1 1600 1 2000	1 Self-Employed 5 Unem-ployed 4 Volunteers	3 Married 2 Widows 1 Separated 4 Single
Focus Group 3 Champi-ons of Christ N= 12	9 Female 3 Male Ages 21-80	24 Relatives 2 Neighbors 7 Friends Ages Indicated 7-54	3 None 3 1000 1 1500 2 2000 2 3000 1 5000	2 Self Employed 3 Employed 1 Volunteer 6 Unem-ployed	3 Married 1 Widow 3 Separated 5 Single
Focus Group 4 St. Michael's N= 11	10 Female 1 Male Ages 25-45	11 Relatives 10 Neighbors 18 Friends Ages indicated 3-28	6 None 1 1000 1 2000 3 3000	1 Self-Employed 2 Employed 2 Volunteers 6 Unem-ployed	3 Married 1 Divorced 3 Widows 4 Single
	N=43	N=116			

Source: HGO Focus Groups, 2006

Chapter 5

CAREGIVER PERSPECTIVES AND CHALLENGES

HIV/AIDS Caregivers Perspective on Caregiver Role

Caregivers in this research open our minds to the extraordinary work that they perform while keeping our attention on the persons and communities that they care for. Their description of daily responsibilities expose us to their concerns about children and widows; those without transportation, housing, food; those facing financial challenges and unemployment; and probably most importantly those facing discrimination and stigmatization that deny them needed treatment and the dignity needed to face another day. The caregivers give us added insight about faith. Many know the scriptural definition of faith as the substance of things hoped for; the evidence of things not seen (Hebrews 11:1). These caregivers have yet to see the full-range of support that they believe is required; yet they have faith that the things they need and hope for will be made available through their sharing their voices.

Collectively, the 43 caregivers are rays of light and hope for the 48 relatives, 47 friends and 21 neighbors. These 116 individuals served are multiplied by the members in their households and the communities where they reside. It is very important to acknowledge that over half (58%) of the caregivers provide support to friends and neighbors. This is indeed a manifestation of Ubuntu.

The authors wish to borrow the sentiments of the 34 women and 9 men and state that their voices represents hearts of hope...and our hearts beat for them and the works they do to make life better for persons with HIV and AIDS.

57

All of the caregiver quotes included in this chapter are the voices of those who participated in the focus group described in Chapter 4.

How individuals respond to situations is often associated with their "outlook" about the situation (Crewe, 2003). The first question posed to the caregiver was to share the first thing that came to mind when they heard the term "HIV/AIDS Caregiver." Table 6 provides an overview of their responses.

Table 6:   HIV/AIDS Caregiver Reaction to Caregiver Responsibilities

Group 1 KARIOBANGI HIV/AIDS Program	*Financial Strain *Extreme Burden *Requires a Godly Heart	*Role of Confidante *Stressful Situation *Hopeful
Group 2 WEMA Center	*Sympathetic to Situation *Sense of Helplessness *Confusion *Counselor	*Empathy towards Patient *Feelings of Isolation *At Risk (exposure to blood)
Group 3 Champions of Christ	*Comfort to Patient *Sense of Helplessness	*Role of Confidant
Group 4 St. Michael Catholic Church HIV/AIDS Support Program	*Giver of Hope *Provides Encouragement *Educator	*Confidante *Showing Love *Being a Friend

Source: HGO Focus Groups, 2006

Table 7: Themes Associated with Caregiver Reaction to Caregiver Responsibilities

Themes Identified	Terms Used
Motivations/Benefits	Comfort to patients
	Giver of hope
	Being a friend
	Showing love
Risks/Burden	Financial strain
	Extreme burden
	Stressful situation
	Profound sacrifice
	Sense of helplessness
	At risk-exposure to blood
Roles/Duties	Role of confidante
	Counselor
	Comfort to patient
	Educator
	Being a friend
Qualities Needed	Requires a Godly heart
	Empathy toward patients
	Provide encouragement
	Showing love
Reactions to Role	Hopeful
	Sympathetic to situation
	Confusion
	Feeling of isolation
	Profound sacrifice
	Sense of helplessness

Source: Authors

Table 8: HIV/AIDS Caregiver Challenges

Group 1 KARIOBANGI HIV/AIDS Program	*Stigma Attached to Role *Gender Concerns *Unemployment *Housing *Insufficient Community Programs	*Lack of Money *Antiseptic Needs *Effects of Meds. On Patients *Transportation (ambu-lance)
Group 2 WEMA Center	* Discrimination *Basic Needs Not Met * High Expectations of Patient * Street Children & Prostitu-tion * Limited Antiseptic Supplies* *Lack of Caregiver Job Skills	*Stigma *Resources for Orphans *Transportation *Finances (rent) *Low Moral *Housing (rent cannot be paid)
Group 3 Champions of Christ	*Financial Strain *Transportation *Perceptions of HIV/AIDS (bewitched) *Lack of Caregiver Training	*Lack of Medication *Unemployment *Stigma Attached to Role
Group 4 St. Michael Catholic Church HIV/AIDS Support Program	*Poverty *Stigmatized *Non acceptance of HIV (patient and family) *Difficult During Rainy Season *Basic Needs of Patient Not Met	*Lack of Resources *Family Requests Caregiver Disclosure *Transportation *Limited Supplies- Medical (i.e. gloves) and antiseptic

Source: HGO Focus Groups, 2006

Caregivers use a range of terms to describe their caregiving responsibilities. The terms describe both positive and negative aspects of caregiving. A closer examination of their choices of words to describe their responsibilities calls attention to their motivations for becoming caregivers, including the benefits, the risks, and their various roles. Their descriptors reveal the complexity in providing care for persons that are infected and affected by HIV and AIDS. Also, the terms provide a glimpse into the realities of being a caregiver and offer a beginning list of qualities needed to deliver services and the role of the caregiver. Table 7 presents these themes.

The themes document that caregivers are motivated by their desire to be of assistance. They do so understanding the risks and burden of financial strain, stress, safety risks, and sacrifices required. They understand that caregivers require empathy and the ability to encourage. Of particular importance are the caregivers' reactions to their self-identified roles of confidante, counselor, educator, and friend. While hopeful and sympathetic, the dominant reactions to the responsibilities were expressed in negative terms such as confusion, isolation, sacrifice, and helplessness. Also, the faith-based organization focus groups clearly use positive words as compared with the other two NGOs that more heavily emphasized the stressors associated with caregiving. This has clear implications for practice that will be discussed later.

Table 8 summarizes the key challenges that were identified by caregivers by focus group affiliation in their discussion about caring for HIV/AIDS infected individuals.

All of the groups identified discrimination and stigma, financial needs/lack of resources, transportation, basic needs of patients, and poverty/unemployment/housing. Although isolated for the purpose of discussion, the challenges were often bundled and demonstrated the complexity of the needs of persons served. Unlike the responses to caregiver responsibilities, the list of challenges were similar among all of the groups---there was no clear pattern that differentiated one group from the other or the faith based vs. NGO groups.

The sections that follow provide greater detail regarding themes that help to understand selected caregiver responsibilities and challenges. Using grounded theory and content analysis, the authors identified themes that emerged from the 17 single spaced pages of transcript. Using the following coding techniques, the themes that are presented emerged to answer the following questions:

1. How do caregivers perceive their roles?
2. What challenges are present as they carry out their caregiving roles?

The following analytic strategies were used to identify themes related to the two key questions.

*   *Coding* is a process for both categorizing qualitative data and for describing the implications and details of these categories.
*   *Memoing* is a process for recording the thoughts and ideas of the researcher as they evolve throughout the study.
*   *Integrative diagrams and sessions* are used to pull all of the detail together to help make sense of the data with respect to the emerging theory (Trochim, 2006).

Caregiving Perspectives: Help, Hope, and Faith

Caregivers are diverse in their thinking and responses to their role as caregivers. Their reactions when asked to address the first thing that comes to mind about caregiving ranges from their feelings about the care receiver to their feelings about their approach to caregiving. Embedded in their responses are statements related to the helping process, hope and faith. Caregiving for them is much greater than meeting the physical needs of the receivers; it is reciprocal and heavily guided by faith and spirituality. The seamless link between the statements of help, hope, and faith necessitate that help, hope, and faith be considered as one holistic theme that directs their actions. The following statements are grouped by the individual themes but are best understood through thinking about them collectively.

Help

- We do have a heart of wanting to help, but when it comes to money matters, it becomes a problem to assist a patient somewhere... but when it comes to encourage verbally the patient gets encouraged, but other than being encouraged, he needs food, clothing, and all types of help, but if you do not have the capacity, you find you are stranded – so our biggest problem is money, and we are asking God to help us.
- The first thing that comes to mind (when hearing the word caregiver) is to help those people.
- Caregiving is something that somebody does at his or her own risk – nobody pay you... you just ask yourself a question... you sympathize but not always sympathizing because we are taught to be always empathetic to them.

Hope

- You tell them (HIV patients) that being sick is not the end of the world.
- You try to be close to the patient so he does not feel neglected.
- You try being close to them so that you can advise them more not to despair even if the children have deserted them, you stick close to them so that they are assured that they are not alone... you are with them voluntarily to visit them and feed.

Faith

- If you don't have a Godly heart you will be tempted to run away from the patient. Since you were used to seeing him walking now he is bed ridden you will have mercy, and it is very painful because you will ask yourself, for sure God loves me but my colleague is sick; that is when you sacrifice whole-heartedly to help because he has not wronged God neither have you and he is bedridden. That is why we have offered ourselves to **help** and there is no remuneration we are given. But we do the service with the purpose of assisting our colleagues since they are bedridden.

- I love my patients, and I always encourage them never to give up because God will help them and they will get well.

- Personally, I feel sympathy [towards] the person who is infected and doesn't have the strength to fend for himself and he is just there – cannot eat. Somebody has to do his utensils and even give water. It is God's love for somebody to sacrifice to assist because this disease did not come because of the wish of the person – it came to the human race and even if maybe not with AIDS everybody will die.

- We always sympathize with them in one way or another, it is one way of preaching to one…sometimes you are stigmatized in your community…they know you have HIV, you are abandoned – so when you decide to be an HIV caregiver, you ask yourself so many questions, but while doing this, you do not want to know who will pay you…we always tell ourselves that it is God who will pay us caregivers of HIV victims

These voices of persons who are caregivers reflect their strong faith and commitment to helping and transmitting hope to persons infected with AIDS. It is very difficult to isolate their caregiving philosophy from their spirituality and spirit of beneficence. While these caregivers were not infected, they are clearly affected and feel it is their destiny to care for and about those with AIDS.

Perspective of Infected Caregivers: Stigmatization and Anger

Another group of caregivers in the study were both infected and affected by HIV/AIDS and their perspectives congregate around feelings of stigma. They are consumed with feelings of being judged individually and collectively for immoral behavior contributing to their illness. Because of these misconceptions, the infected caregiver is cast as being responsible for the illness rather than a victim. Often, this invokes anger. The caregivers below reflect the tension of being a caregiver yet coping with the illness oneself.

- The thing that I've seen openly – especially us suffering from this disease of AIDS and those who are HIV positive...the truth is that when people see you emaciated you don't have the strength to walk – when they see you, they start talking about you...this person looks like he is infected.
- What I think when people hear HIV/AIDS? They always think that the only people that have this disease are prostitutes...not knowing that it is a disease that comes just as you, a mother, you are in the house and you do not know what your man went out and had or did but you as a faithful mother in the house doing your household chores and in the long run you find yourself having AIDS.

Stress and Sacrifice

In addition to the voices of the caregivers about their positive motivation toward helping, is the underlying stress that accompanies their help, hope, and faith. It was more clearly heard from the caregivers that they were facing personal hardships as they carried out their responsibilities and trying to meet the needs of families and communities affected with HIV and AIDS. Although the section that follows characterizes challenges discussed by the caregivers, the literature is clear about the differentiation between challenges and stressors. According to Germain and Gitterman (1995)

> Life stressors and challenges differ in meaning and emotional tone. A stressor represents serious harm or loss and is associated with a sense of being in jeopardy. A challenge is experienced as an opportunity for growth and is associated with positive feelings and anticipated mastery and zestful struggle (p. 817).

The voices of the caregivers expose us to the stressors that they are experiencing because of poverty and oppression. This is particularly evident as they speak about the need to sacrifice to provide care. The following comment from a caregiver about women is particularly relevant to the observation that women are often left behind to provide the care.

- Caregiving is a sacrifice, mostly fathers die first then the women...so women are the people that are left behind, and our society believes that women should not work – they should sit in the house and wait for the husband to provide...mostly our husbands are the sole breadwinners.

As you read the words of caregivers, you will hear the multiple stressors that result in feelings of guilt, anxiety, anger, and fear. Prolonged stress with ineffective coping can lead to social dysfunction (Germain and Gitterman). While there is evidence of prolonged stress among caregivers, they seem to have protective factors that keep them grounded and focused—thus the authors have chosen challenges to describe their experiences. As noted by Germain and Gitterman, a "challenge may stir up periodic anxiety, but the person continues to feel hopeful and confident and maintain relatedness, a sense of competence, self-esteem and self-direction" (p. 817). Using this as a frame of reference, the following sections, explore ten challenges in their roles as caregivers. The ten challenges that are presented are related to: 1) Impact on children, 2) financial hardships, 3) food, clothing, shelter, and transportation; 4) widowhood, 5) stigmatization and discrimination, 6) employment, 7) safety, 8) treatment, 9) training and support, 10) advocacy. Finally, the voices reflect upon the importance of support groups in addressing their challenges and possible self-care.

Caregiver Voices and Challenges Faced

Impact on Children –I am Pleading on Behalf of the Children

Perhaps one of the greatest tragedies of the HIV/AIDS pandemic is its impact on children. The caregivers emphasized that the future of the children is being compromised by the family instability they face as a result of parents who are infected. Additionally, a number of children are also infected. When a parent has HIV/AIDS, the children often have to fend for themselves and become adults before their time. Children face hunger, homelessness, a disruption in education, and a general sense of vulnerability and loss. HIV/AIDS orphaned children face life with uncertainty and sometimes engage in risky behavior to survive. The caregivers in this study address the following challenges facing children: Housing and Food; *School Attendance; Risky Behavior; and Mental Well-Being.*

Housing and Food:

- There is the problem of street children, who end up in the streets after their parents have died (from AIDS) – all they need is a good shelter, food and to be able to go to school…so I am pleading on behalf of the street children
- I've been a caregiver since the year 2003 and in most cases, I get interested in the children because once I hear there is a sick person somewhere, the first person my heart beats for is the child because if it is the mother who is sick in that family or the father this child is affected in very

many ways – most of them drop out of school…when they wake up, the house is in confusion; there is no food, and they cannot go to school on empty stomachs. Perhaps most of them opt to sit at home. There is no care in that family. You find the child has got nobody to look after him.

School Attendance

- Some of them (children) are very bright and have not reported to school and at the same time, some of them are caregivers.
- There are these children who have dropped out of school because of school fees, HIV pandemic, early marriage, early pregnancy…a child having a child. If we can have these
- centers where these children can really be looked after…honestly, we should be creating employment for our Country and at the same time caring for our own citizens instead of leaving the children to roam the street.

Risky Behavior

- If they (children) are getting to adolescent stage, you find that this is the time that children opt to go to the streets…some of them start practicing early sex because we know they want to get incentives of what they cannot get from their sick parents.
- We tried (caregivers), the government has tried to remove the street children, but it is hard to wipe out the problem because when these children are left on their own, all they try to do is to fend on their own by scavenging on the street to get something, and the problem is very rampant here in Dandor, and with the dumping site (garbage), we don't know what to do but to pray to God.

Mental Well-Being

Being homeless and hungry is a terrible plight for any person and even more especially children. Equally important is the lack of knowledge about why their lives are being turned upside down. Caregivers expressed concern about children who are facing this disruption without benefit of knowing that their parents are infected with HIV/AIDS. This compounds their trauma, and caregivers find themselves faced with the ethical dilemma of sharing or keeping the family secret. One caregiver stated:

> Children from such families (HIV/AIDS) at times their parents don't even tell them that they are sick – the children just see people lying in bed not knowing what they are suffering from...the children are in a dilemma, not knowing how to be helped not even knowing where the father was working to be assisted for payment or if the mother was doing business – does she have [a] mother anywhere?

Every caregiver expressed concern about the children. The concern is both present and futuristic. Given the pandemic, there is the underlying concern that the children who survive will be able to properly develop so that they can become healthy adults and assume the challenges necessary for them to steer the next generation through the crisis. It is very clear that the impact on children is inextricably linked to the way forward.

Financial Challenges – A Heart to Help

The financial challenges of receiving quality health care are not unique to HIV AIDS infected persons. Unfortunately, too many households suffer from the dual impact of illness and financial worries. The lack of money is inextricably linked to the impact that the illness has on the family. For families who were already experiencing financial hardships or those who have a fragile system of economic support, the impact of HIV/AIDS is compounded, and indeed the lack of financial support may be the tipping point between living and dying. Also, caregivers are in the mix of the financially fragile. They too are struggling and find themselves not only in the caregiving role but in the financial support role. This dual relationship adds to the stress of caregivers, yet it telegraphs a message about the ordinary persons, who provide extraordinary care and support to the loved ones, friends, neighbors, and unrelated fellow human beings. The following statements made by caregivers reinforce the impact of financial challenges on both the caregiver and the care receiver.

- The mother who does a small business of making dough-nuts by the side of the road…people are shunning from buying from her because her skin is rough – the father, who cannot work sends the children to school to be given food…so the little I have I got to share with them.

- In most cases, you get to know that they have not even eaten the whole day. Since the neighbors or even the rela-tives do not near the patient's place, so even when you go there, you do not even have a job, but you have a heart to help – you will use all your resources and money at your disposal.

- The problem we are facing is that when you get in touch or be with the patient, they believe you have come with this money to assist her or him – you have come with the hope, which they believe you are a **heart of hope** to him and actually when you go there maybe you've gone for spiritual assistance; you've counseled her, and he or she finds out that you are just there; you are not helping them in any way as a caregiver (financial), you'll have to dip in-to your pocket to save the situation.

- There are a lot of challenges – the person who has been abandoned has got nothing to eat, but you can even sacri-fice from your own pocket the little you have; you might not even be having an income, but you feel whatever little that you have you share with the victim.

- At times we (caregivers) end up contributing; last week we were here and three of our patients were down, and we could not come to see them empty handed…hence, we contributed twenty, thirty shillings and gave…to those of us to go see them…the biggest challenge is finance.

These statements affirm that the financial challenges are not just visited upon the care receivers, but the care providers are experiencing the strain of wanting to help and being left to do this incredible work with resources of the heart. The relationships of NGOs will be discussed later in the book; however, it is clear that there is a political aspect associated with the financial challenge. The following words from a caregiver make this point.

- We the caregivers cannot actually say we have a source of income where we can base in order to help the community – the people in need don't have the education to know that we are helping, especially those suffering from HIV and AIDS; they believe there is money to be given to them for assistance in each and every problem they are facing, but you find that it is a problem for we caregivers to access those funds, as they believe that we got donors, we got NGOs who have money for this pandemic.

The caregivers remind us that in the war to save persons and families infected and affected by HIV AIDS, often caring is not enough. Dr. Martin Luther King, Nobel Peace Prize recipient, has a line in his world famous, "I Have A Dream" speech that seems to uniquely address the situation. He proclaimed that America had written African Americans a check that was returned for "insufficient funds" because of its failure to render social and economic justice (King, 1986). The caregivers identify with the importance of aligning financial resources and social justice with the persons who are providing and receiving care. The failure to do so, as stated by the caregivers, has the unintended consequence of diminishing the caregiver in the eyes of the care receiver.

Clearly there is a need to provide needed financial support to the hearts of hope that make personal sacrifices to support at the micro and macro levels.

Food, Clothing, Shelter, and Transportation Challenges - Today You Go Empty Handed

Maslov (1943) introduced the importance of meeting physiological and safety needs before self-actualization could occur. Included in these two lower level needs are food and shelter. Additionally, transportation is also a security need because it is the bridge between life and death for persons who need treatment. Caregivers provide a clear understanding of the necessity of meeting these basic needs in their work. The caregivers focus extensively on the importance of food to the well-being of the care receivers as well as themselves. The caregivers made 15 specific references to food deprivation. The following observations document the importance given to food, clothing, shelter, and transportation.

- When we go to that house, there is no food; basically, the needs that are essential to the family [are] not there – We are forced to dig in our pockets and get something to assist.
- There is the problem of street children, who end up in the streets after their parents have died (from AIDS) – all they need is a good shelter, food, and to be able to go to school…so I am pleading on behalf of the street children.
- The main challenges we face on the ground, when you go to visit a patient you yourself, you are not paid…but they expect you to take them food, medicines, and so forth – on medicines there are some organizations that are giving like the Maltissa, but when it comes to food, it is a big problem. Since once they have taken their antiviral they want to eat so well…today you go empty handed and the following day the same – the patient will not even want to

look at you, in fact some refuse even talking to you...and you are like bothering them, going empty handed.

- Most of the money we've been spending comes from our own pockets, but once in a while from close relatives or well-wishers...when my friends hear there is somebody who is sick or I am helping, they help me with something small – If we talk as a group when we decide to go visit a patient, we decide to contribute as a group...when we are in church, we talk to the worshippers – those who can help us to lend a hand with things like clothes, food – basically these are the donations we've been relying on.

- When I am in the field the whole day...I get nothing and my children, in the afternoon, they want to eat and I've got nothing to give them. If at least I could be getting something small, it will be fine.

Like food and clothing, housing is also considered by caregivers as extremely important to quality of life. The reference to housing was often inextricably linked to the financial hardship experienced as a result of HIV and AIDS. One caregiver states:

- Another thing, these people live in rented houses, and the owner may not allow them to live for two or three months without paying them...he locks them out – as a caregiver, when you go and find your patient and children locked out of the house you do [not] know who to go and face – the only alternative is to go to the local Chief who gives you a letter to come and plead with the owner of the house to be allowed in...but who is going to pay the outstanding rent?

Transportation is also identified by caregivers as a barrier to needed assistance. The lack of transportation is also associated with stigma. This statement from a caregiver explains this.

- Another problem we are facing – we work in the slums, and there are patients who cannot walk to the main road, and when you approach a person for assistance, they want money, and the issue of transportation in the interior you have to use a bicycle from the interior to the main road to get a minibus and at times the owners of minibuses do not want to carry patients; hence, we are stranded and at times we go to the local Chief Camp or Elders to contribute some money; we hire a vehicle to take the patients to Mbagathi District Hospital or Kenyatta National Hospital for treatment. Therefore, transport is a major problem to us.

• If somebody can buy us an ambulance…we don't have an ambulance in Dandora, and most of the times you find people carried on hand cart, being taken to the hospital – we are forced to go door to door trying…raising money to dash a sick patient to Kenyatta National Hospital.

Widowhood Challenges - Now Who Will Help Them?

The challenges faced by widows/widowers are actually a subset of the financial challenges just discussed. Yet widowhood was mentioned so often that it warranted a separate discussion. Grief and loss accompany most illnesses. However, when the loss of a spouse has the added impact of financial strain and stigma associated with death, the widow or widower is profoundly impacted. Of course, the impact of the loss is related to the strength of the relationship before the death, as well as the roles carried out by each spouse. As caregivers examined the impact of widowhood, they clearly understood the complexity of gender roles and cultural expectations of the husband or the wife. What seems most revealing in the comments related to widowhood is the lack of attention to the grief process—it can be surmised that survival crowds out the needed grieving process. This is yet another dimension of how normal and necessary processes to maintain emotional wellbeing are removed from many as they face the challenges associated with living or dying with HIV/AIDS. The words of the caregivers expose the pain associated with the loss of a spouse.

- If your husband has died, there is nobody who will take responsibility of your upkeep unless you yourself derive a way of your survival together with your children to make your family unit strong. Widows really face it rough – I am pleading for the sake of the widows, especially those who were housewives and the husbands were the ones who used to work. Now the husband has died, and they don't have a rough idea on how to cope with life because they were dependent on their husbands to bring home milk, food, and everything...now, who will help them? Not neighbors, nor the relatives; therefore, widows have a big, big problem.

- In a situation where you have lost a husband and you are left behind with five children or seven or so forth, you find a situation where relatives are discriminating, rejecting, and not considering your children as one of them...you find a widow is down; the children are desperate – nobody is willing to provide for them; the children go to the street...even the in-laws don't care for them- that is the greatest problem we face.

Although most of the comments were directed toward widows, men who have lost their wives also suffer greatly. Like women, the cultural responsibilities shift when the spouse is no longer in the family. The care of children is an example of the added responsibility that the husband faces. When one adds to the equation that he too is infected, the realities are even more overwhelming. The tragic overlay of stigmatization is clearly articulated by a caregiver in the following statement.

- I've got a patient, [whose] wife died, and the husband is surviving; he's undergone so much...nobody wanted to help him – not even his own brother until his small children had to help their father; he has really suffered to the extent that he is refusing to take medicine so that he dies fast. I went and talked to him and tried convincing him to take the drugs, but he is refusing to eat – therefore, we got a big problem…and the neighbors when you go to clean his beddings, they don't want you to pour the remains in the toilet (thinking) that you will infect them – they don't greet him or even want to meet him on the way or share a toilet with him…HIV patients really suffer.

Widowhood also has an unforgiving impact on the lives of children that find themselves having to step in for family members that are unable or unwilling to help. The tragedy of this is that financial necessity sometimes pushes children into lifestyles that place them at risk. Also, the burden of a "childless" childhood is very likely to have a lifetime impact on their quality of life and well-being. While not specifically stated, the caregivers are most likely providing the children with a glimpse of humanity in what must seem like an uncaring world.

Stigmatization and Misinformation Challenges - Nobody Values You

United Nations Secretary-General Ban Ki Moon Washington Times (Aug 6, 2008) says:

"Stigma remains the single most important barrier to public action. It is a main reason why so many people are afraid to see a doctor to determine whether they have the disease, or to seek treatment if so. It helps make AIDS the silent killer because people fear the social disgrace of speaking about it, or of taking easily available precautions. Stigma is a chief reason why the AIDS epidemic continues to devastate societies around the world." Caregivers in this research agree that persons with HIV and AIDS experience prejudices and discrimination that multiplies their suffering. Managing their illness is compounded by the downward glances of the community and most notably the disengagement of the extended family that is so much a part of the Kenyan culture.

Stigmatization is not easily isolated from the other aspects of caregiver perspectives about HIV and AIDS. It seems to be embedded in other challenges, and the authors isolate it to draw attention to its power on the various layers of the ecological system. As with many of the themes, the caregiver is a source of care and also in need of care. Caregivers too have taken on the burden of stigma and discrimination that penetrates the systems of care. Like most stigmas, fear of HIV and AIDS is inextricably woven into the fabric of a community that is sometimes inadequately informed and other times inadequately protected from the pandemic. The caregivers below describe their first hand exposure to the prejudices, negative attitudes, and maltreatment that is placed on *both the caregiver and receiver of care.*

- When somebody is abandoned and you volunteer yourself to go care for him/her
- you do not expect anything or anyone is coming to pay you unless somebody comes to your rescue...there are so many things you put into consideration – you go there, you take care of the person who is HIV positive, and nobody cares even that the home is being isolated because they think if that person [has] HIV and even by greeting you...you can be infected.
- There are our neighbors who are infected, and there are those who don't want to see him or like him, and they have a tendency of insulting them...so the patient takes it that nobody values him, even his family – the parents insult him and chase him away...so he decides he better go and steal and if he will be killed, especially if caught stealing, will be the solution to leave this misery...since even his friends don't wanna see him." (response from a teen-age caregiver)
- Your colleague, your sister, and even your mother when they realize you are HIV positive, they don't treat you like a human being – you are deserted.

In addition to the stigma and discrimination that the care receivers feel from the outside world, is the concern that the caregiver will violate their confidentiality by sharing their circumstances with the community. The following caregiver quote expresses this concern.

- The problem that we are actually facing on the ground with HIV and AIDS, we hear that caregivers are working to take care of these people living with HIV and AIDS. The first thing in their minds is that their names will be told to others in the community, but the whole society knows, so they fear the caregivers coming to their houses and taking care of them.

Among the most vulnerable casualties of stigma and discrimination are children who must live in a world that rejects them. The voices of the caregivers quoted below are particularly poignant about the children, who bear the weight of stigma and discrimination.

- We need information centers, schools for the school going children – hospitals, and dispensaries where they can go and be treated nicely without [any] discrimination. We need to have a place where they can play as children.
- …their small child, who is seven years old and who has skin rashes…in school, his fellow children refuse to sit next to him, telling him that he is infecting with the skin disorder.

Additionally, caregivers expressed the need for education to prevent stigma. These voices explicate the value-based assumptions surrounding the families that bear the burden of HIV and AIDS. Further, they extended their concern regarding the need for educators to address stigmatization and discrimination. For example, they stated

- The people who are not suffering do not accept the patients because in our African set up, they believe AIDS comes because of witchcraft...so the first challenge we face is people who are not suffering to accept those who are HIV [positive].

- So many people tend to speculate on the disease as witch-craft, and yet you see this person is sick...but because of lack of information to know that this person is sick, and the lack of enough personnel to go out there and talk about HIV/AIDS, so many people who we are with in schools and even church...so many of them do not know about HIV/AIDS, so they don't have the right information.

- We started an outreach by telling the people around us on open forums how the world is now...not necessarily tell-ing them that we are infected, but to stand up like heroes and fight this deadly disease; who knows, most of us will start being open and follow us who stood to talk and share about the patients they have been hiding.

- The main problem we face as caregivers – people do not have the right information...they depend on what they hear in the neighborhood – groups of people talking...they do not have the correct information concerning HIV/AIDS – and because of that, they place themselves in compro-mising behaviors that are risky to their lives and even those who are sick do not know if they are sick because they do not understand.

As caregivers discuss stigma and discrimination, they bring attention to the inhumanity of the HIV/AIDS pandem-ic. They use their understanding to tell their story and advo-cate for an approach that addresses the misinformation in the community as well as the opportunity to empower in-fected and affected persons to use their person to give voice to solutions.

Employment Challenges - They're In a Fix

Like the other themes presented by caregivers, the dialogue about employment intersects other pressing concerns. The caregivers spoke about their own employment challenges, as

well as the challenges of the persons in their care. Of particular importance is their reference to lack of employment and
children living on the street. Caregivers stated

- In most cases people are jobless [and surviving by] selling
  vegetables by the roadside and have saved something for
  their children...by the time they are down and bedridden
  the children have got nobody to care for them or feed
  them, hence they end up on the street and that has contributed to the number of street children in Kenya today.
- The moment the person is known to be HIV, he cannot
  work or his earnings drop...so these people tend to depend
  on the caregivers, who some of them cannot even afford to
  support themselves medical, hence, economically because
  of the setup of our country...you live by the sweat of your
  own hands, and working with your hands, you need to use
  a lot of energy and these people are suffering. Therefore,
  you find that they're in a fix when it comes to their earn-
  ing because they cannot work as hard as before.
- Concerning this AIDS disease...I am an employer of one
  of the patients, I try visiting so many patients, but the idea
  is tough because so many do not accept their situation because of the fear of being despised by their relatives and
  shunned out...life can be hard if somebody is employed –
  if he mentions he is infected, he can be retired or where he
  lives nobody dares to visit him.

As stated, the caregivers also reflected on their lack of
employment (income), and how it impacts their ability to
support both the persons cared for and themselves.

- The problem which is there with these patients when it
  reaches a point where a person has taken anti-viral which
  are very powerful – they have effects of somebody vomit-
  ing; his legs lacking strength – so you see this is a very
  tough time when you go there you don't have a job. You
  try pleading with your family to give you some food to
  bring to the patient [but] when you give him the food he

vomits, hence having nothing to sustain him in the stomach, so you wonder what to do.

- Most of us are not employed, some of us, as you can see...we used to be fat – some of us had husbands but were separated, so having some savings somewhere can be a problem...if it's children, you find you feed them with what you have, but when it comes to money issues, it becomes a problem...say you have to assist somebody with 1,000 shillings and back at your home you have not eaten or fed...you have to consider yourself.
- Poverty...these sides we have a problem of income – therefore, getting food and clothing to patients who do not have...they expect us as caregivers taking care of them to provide.

The strengths perspective in social work requires attention to resilience and the resourcefulness within persons, who are faced with challenges. The voices of caregivers affirmed the strengths of the caregivers and their ability to help without sustained employment or pay.

- That is we have offered ourselves to help, and there is no remuneration we are given. But we do the service with the purpose of assisting our colleagues since they are bedridden.
- If we can get First Aid kits, soap, antiseptics, towels, basins because at times you enter somebody's house, and he or she has got nothing to use, and that is a big challenge – so you go there and get a relative; when you ask for some soap, he or she says they don't have...you have to dip into your own pocket to buy soap, and at times when you talk to the patients, they tell you they cannot hear because of feeling dizzy since they have not eaten – then you have to go or send somebody to buy a quarter kilogram of sugar to prepare porridge for the patient, and before you go, [you have] to leave them with something....
- We all know that these patients at any minute they can get serious...and when the disease sparks off, they cannot

walk, and therefore, you look for ways of dashing them to the hospital, therefore, you have to think fast, and if you book for a taxi, you have to pay for it.

The caregivers provide insight on the challenges related to employment, and how the lack of employment/income hinders their ability to deliver the best quality care. However, the caregivers demonstrate their willingness to use their own resources despite their own lack of employment. The discussion surrounding caregiving is paramount in understanding that the caregiver and care receiver boundaries are extremely permeable.

Safety Challenges - Risking Your Own Life

Caregivers understand that they are sometimes at risk when they provide the needed care to persons with AIDS. Despite the risks, they serve. Interestingly, this was not a dominant theme. This can reasonably be attributed to their faith and passion to serve. Thus, attention to risks was secondary to other areas that focused more on the needs of the persons being cared for and about.

- At times, the house is in a mess and some of them cannot even make [it] to the toilet…hence, finishing their business on the bedding…you will have to clean, and at times, you don't have gloves – we end up using polythene papers. You enter their house; they have not cleaned them, and there is no soap or any detergent – you end up using cheap soap, which is not effective…hence, you are also risking you own life because who knows, you can also get infection in the process…but because you have a willing heart, you end up doing it.
- Those (caregivers) visiting patients, if they could get First Aid kits, gloves, detergent, medicine, it would be helpful…because caregivers are scared of putting a risk on their own lives by using polythene bags.

While only a few caregivers specifically mentioned health risks, others explained their work, and the nature of their work documents their exposure.

- A person like me, when I got to take care of somebody who is bedridden, you find that person sleeping on the side – you have to change the patient on the other side, you have to wash the patient, and if you have no sympathy, you cannot do such a thing.

It is clear that risks to health are accepted by caregivers. It is most likely considered necessary to carry out the calling to help. Sometimes the caregivers request items to protect themselves from exposure. What is equally apparent is their exposure to stress and mental anguish and its potential toll on their well-being and quality of life.

Treatment Challenges and Approaches - Nothing is too Hard to Bear

Caregivers recognize that effective treatment is multifaceted. Accessibility, affordability, and cultural awareness are necessary conditions for optimal treatment. The caregivers also voice challenges associated with the person's ability to accept his or her condition and the concern about confidentiality. Also, treatment outcomes are related to other factors such as availability of food. Food deprivation is a deterrent to treatment, and caregivers recognize the need to address this.

- The patients when they are on antiviral [medicine], they really want to eat properly and without eating properly, they perish early…and the medicines are strong and cannot be taken without food. Others even default after realizing that they don't have food, and the aftermath of the drugs is powerful – they tremble and cannot even walk and become weak…so they refuse to take the medicines.

Similarly, the importance of being culturally aware and sensitive is important to caregivers and their ability to provide effective treatment. The following statement captures this.

- The time they are very weak they cannot even manage to support themselves out there, so there is need to match the sex – I mean maybe the caregiver is a woman and the sick person is a man....now, there is a problem. On the other hand, you find that the one who is sick does not want to see even a woman coming to attend to him because he is afraid of [exposing] his private areas, and the same applies to the female – this has brought a lot of problems to caregivers.

For treatment to be successful, caregivers ascribe importance to the patient's ability to accept his or her diagnosis. According to caregivers, this is a problem.

- Another problem is that there are some of them who do not want to accept their situation.
- Those who have accepted themselves, that they are sick, it is easy to reach them and make the work of a caregiver more bearable...they come to talk to you and seek counseling.

Caregivers are dispensers of hope. Their approach to treatment is greatly influenced by their faith and spirituality. They are motivated by their beliefs that they have a spiritual obligation to serve. This is one of the most recurring themes. There were 15 direct references to God. The following quotes document how God is integrated into their philosophy of treatment.

- People suffering from the HIV have a different kind of disease, especially our fellow women when we go to bathe them...and if you don't love God and have a joy of salvation, you can never work for people who are bedridden and especially suffering from AIDS.

- So many of us think [the only way] you get the HIV/AIDS is through sex, but through how we have been educated and the way we've read a lot, we know you can get this disease even if you have not slept with anybody...I for example, if I tell people that I am infected and yet I am saved, they insult me and ask me – then how come I got the disease? It becomes a struggle in me...but because I trust in God, I take heart and even to those who talk ill I tell them, "this is something that can also get you, and you will start looking for me for advice" – all I insist on telling them is to continue waiting upon God because in each and everything that happens, God usually has his purpose...so we should not feel that we are weak like the way we visit people and they insult us and some even not impressed with our presence, but still they've not agreed because when they are out there and they hear one has died because of the disease all we need to do, and is possible, is to be courageous...things are tough, but once you are in the Lord...nothing is hard to bear.

Caregiver Training Challenges - Caught Up in the Circumstances

The caregivers from Kenya, like others, did not plan their destiny. For a variety of reasons, mostly related to faith and kinship ties, they find themselves making personal sacrifices to serve the families and individuals who have to turn outward for help. The qualifications seem to be largely a "willing heart," and through limited assistance from NGOs and faith-based organizations, they go about helping in their own ways. Despite the absence of formal preparation, these indigenous caregivers make a difference in the lives of persons, who find themselves sometimes looking to strangers to assist them. The caregivers speak about the limits of their assistance without adequate preparation and support.

- We as caregivers…most of us finding ourselves as care-givers was not out of our own liking; we did not start as caregivers, but we found ourselves in a situation that we were taking care of these people because we are caught up in the circumstances with them – although we help and as-sist them, at times we are stranded on what to do because we are not trained to keep them well and assist them well, but it has become our responsibility to help them.

- If we can be able to be trained and taught well with the right information on the people we visit and talk to…so that we take care of them and ask to protect ourselves, we can be people of great assistance…the people that we help, when they hear that we are not just helping them haphazardly, but we are informed and educated, they will build confidence towards us.

- We would like to have demonstrating materials to educate our children on how to protect themselves (contracep-tives).

- Like me, what I face on the ground…I deal with vulnera-ble and orphan children, and in the place they are staying, they are divided not to share sanitation– at times when they leave their utensils on the sink, they are told never to leave their utensils there but have them in their houses be-cause if they look at that family, the whole of it is suffer-ing from HIV and that is the father, mother, and two children – so they were crying in anguish, and I was won-dering how to help them.

Consistent with other persons who find themselves in caregiver roles, they experience ethical dilemmas. Without formal training, they make mistakes that are charged to their heads and not to their hearts. The following caregiver de-scribes such an ethical dilemma.

- As a caregiver, I remember in 1999 my brother was sick at Kenyatta Hospital (in Nairobi) but not so down – when I was told by the doctor to tell him who I was I told him the sick man is my younger brother. The doctor had already talked to the wife, but she looked weak; he could not tell the wife what he wanted to tell me or my brother, who was sick. So when I went to see him he told me your brother is infected (with HIV) and although he is sick, you should find a way of informing the wife of which I did not do. The mistake that I did was not telling my in-law, who in fact died before my brother…on the other hand, the lady was suffering and nobody knew what it was, and during those days, I felt that it is not good to tell her and up to today, I have a conviction that if maybe I would have told her she wouldn't have died early – so as caregivers, we have some people we hold in confidence and when we are given such messages today it is good to tell them." (He is currently a caregiver for his nephew).

The caregivers in the research recognize that they go beyond the boundaries of patient caregiver relationships. They are sometimes faced with situations that professionals would walk away from, yet they stay and use their mother wit to make the best situations possible in the circumstances.

- Some patients when you take them to the hospital, there are bills to be paid and the relatives have isolated him……so he follows you to assist to settle the bill, and furthermore, if a patient dies in your custody it becomes another problem.
- A patient's condition may get serious at night – and it is hard to say, but some die that same night, and it becomes a problem for you who [has] been taking care for him or her to take them to the morgue since you do not have his proper records or his relatives either…so it becomes hard for you to know where to start if you have no proper information.
- At times, it is very difficult to teach them… how to believe…and yet you gossip about a certain patient on how he is faring in front of them.

Caregivers clearly document their interest in providing the best care possible. They do not wish to be limited by the lack of training and resources. Their words call attention to the dilemmas they face and the possible benefit of more training. It is very important to recognize that their advocacy is for the care receiver and that the emphasis is not self-centered. While they would clearly benefit from the support they identified; it is extraordinary work that they perform given the limited preparation.

Advocacy – We've Got People Suffering on the Ground

In a resounding voice, the caregivers used their knowledge of needs and gaps in resources to express their concern. They clearly articulated the need for systemic improvements to the treatment and care for families experiencing distress due to the devastating effects of HIV and AIDS. They spoke with purpose and passion about what they perceived was "fixable" in the system of care. Their sense of a dispassionate system is evidenced by these statements:

- When you go to organizations, they look down on you...like from which part of mother earth did you surface from?
- People who are not suffering are not concerned about people suffering.
- We've got so many conferences that have been held, so many workshops – these workshops if only they have been held, if we had a resource center all the finances that we are using to attend these in five star hotels, we can use to help people living with HIV and AIDS and so forth – this meeting you could have held it at Serena Hotel – these are big places which it would mean to pay a lot of money and we've got people suffering on the ground.

Caregivers understand that their work alone is not sufficient to address the pandemic. Thus, they expressed frustration with the approaches being used by some of the formal helping systems. Being on the ground and seeing the suffering causes them to express concern about what they perceive at best as systemic apathy and at worst as contempt and lack of caring and concern for those who are suffering. By way of contrast, the caregivers also recognized a few organizations that were indeed assisting them with their work and building their capacity to work more effectively.

> • After talking to an organization called WEMA, they gave us (teenage caregivers) courage to go talk to the patients and bring them closer to reality, urge them to take medicine....and the little we contribute as the youth, we buy them food, clothing…at least they look OK, but back in the home community, they don't walk peacefully – even when a girl sees him, he cannot even go to church, they are insulted, but we and the mothers guide and share ideas with them and have fellowship with them.

Caregivers seemingly accept the resources that are offered and use them to enhance the quality of life of the persons that they serve. While critical of the lack of resources, they continue to look for solutions and do not give up hope. This may be indicative of a need for attention to be given to the self-care of the caregivers. Their comments describe circumstances that are very stressful. Caregiving literature is replete with the call for caregivers to receive respite or self-care. The circumstances alluded to in the following comments support the need for self-care advocacy.

> • At times, you want to go visit a patient and it has rained heavily… mud is everywhere, and there is no way you can step on awful places and you are bare footed.
> • In a day we sleep only four hours, and the remaining twenty we utilize to serve the patients.
> • At times, it is very difficult for the patients to accept you, especially the fact that you were going to take care of them – we counsel them and give them care……..when

you give them drugs, they are furious on why are you giving them drugs when they can take care of themselves......they claim.

Caregivers face death and dying every day. With this,
comes a need to self-reflect and replenish. Thus, self-care
will be an important aspect of the way forward. The discussion that follows on support groups provides preliminary
evidence of the therapeutic value of attention to the caregivers' mental well-being.

Support Groups-What We Mostly Do is Group Therapy

Caregivers speak very positively about the importance of
support groups. Like most support groups, the focus is on
resource sharing as well as an opportunity to share stresses
in a safe place where others understand your passion to help.
The following comments from caregivers describe the value
they attribute to participating in a group. For some the
comments represent their experience in a support group and
for others, the comments are anticipatory.

- You get knowledge and skills from other support groups –
  if the problem they are facing is transportation, with our
  group food and another medicine, maybe by brainstorming
  together we come up with one conclusion.
- Through support groups we've learned that patients are
  really open – the advantages of meeting with other support
  groups they tell you the problems they've been facing, and
  you tell them yours and you exchange ideas.
- The idea of starting a support group for caregivers really
  boosts morale...because you share with your neighbors or
  good Samaritans, who know this is a catastrophe that continues destroying people. There are those people who have
  money, and some of us are still struggling...when you tell
  some people, they insult you, but those who insult you are
  those who do not know who God is...and they do not

know that maybe, one day…they might also get the disease.

- The support group I'm in is to help one another on how we can go and visit others, but we have not gotten assistance as such…but how we help one another, for instance somebody has a patient somewhere; therefore, we brainstorm on what ways to assist the patient, but what we do mostly is a group therapy – we talk together, brainstorm, and also help one another.
- Since we started this support group, we've seen ourselves progressing…whenever we sit down, we share how each one of us can help another.

Support groups seem to be very useful to the caregivers. They seem to value the camaraderie and find renewed strength and resources to deliver needed services. Equally important, support groups expand their capacity to serve through building confidence and providing a platform for them to see themselves progressing in the important work of caregivers.

Chapter 6

THEORETICAL PERSPECTIVES: CAREGIVER
CHALLENGES AND STRENGTH

The authors have chosen the Ecological Systems Theory and Role Theory to explain factors impacting the lives of HIV/AIDS Caregivers.

Ecological Systems Theory

The Ecological Systems Theory explains that individuals are constantly communicating with others and other "systems" in the environment; these systems reciprocally influence each other (Hepworth, Rooney, & Larsen, 1997). Assessment from an ecological perspective requires knowledge of the systems involved in interaction between individuals and their environment (Turner, 1996). The systems include: subsystems of the individual; interpersonal systems; organizations, institutions, and communities; and the physical environment (Hepworth, Rooney, & Larsen, 1997). HIV/AIDS caregivers often use interpersonal systems as resources and have to interact with the following systemic levels identified by Bonfenbrenner's socio cultural view of the person in relationship to environment. Also, Figure 3 depicts the ecological model.

- *Microsystem*- The most basic system, referring to an individual's most immediate environment (i.e., the effects of personality characteristics on other family members).
- *Mesosystem*- A more generalized system, referring to the interactional processes between multiple microsystems (i.e., effects of spousal relationships on parent-child interactions).

- *Exosystem-* Settings on a more generalized level, which affect indirectly, family interactions on the micro and meso levels (i. e., the effects of parent's employment on family interactions).
- *Macrosystem-* The most generalized forces, affecting individuals and family functioning (i.e., political, cultural, economical, and social).
- *Chronosystem-* the patterning of environmental events and transitions over the life course.

Figure 4: Ecological Theory

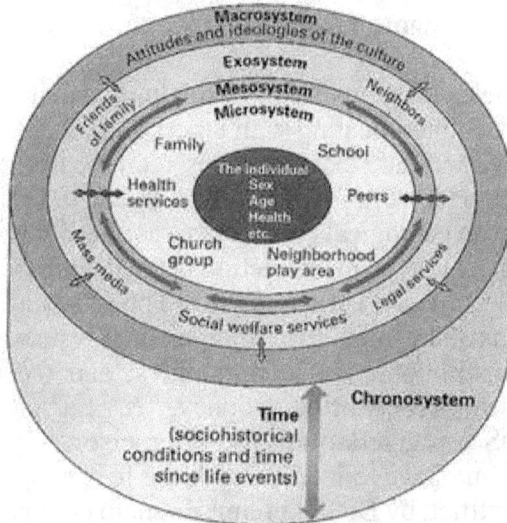

(Brofenbrenner's Ecological Model, 2011)

The ecological theory also helps us to understand that over the life course, individuals and families experience unique developmental pathways. Gitterman (1996) suggests that "over the life course, people strive to improve the level of fit with their environments"

(pp. 390). When we feel positive about our own capacities and hopeful about having our needs and aspirations fulfilled, and when we view our environmental resources as responsive, we and our immediate environments are likely to achieve a reciprocally sustaining condition of adaptability (Gitterman, 1996). Adequate coping resources (formal and informal) are needed to help the caregivers successfully continue their role. Providing resources that are physically accessible to HIV/AIDS caregivers and are within their personal environment could improve their level of fit.

Ecological systems theory provides social workers with a conceptual framework that shifts attention away from a cause-effect relationship between two variables: a person and situation as an interrelated whole. Andrae (1996) suggests that we need to study the entire system in order to understand the dynamic interactions, transactions, and organizational patterns that are critical to the functioning of both the individual and situation (Andrae, 1996).

Numerous Africans view family as a vital part of survival, as evidenced throughout the early historical experience of African people. This powerful ancestral lineage is the backbone and support of a number of African family systems. Working together as a holistic unit is an emphatic value of African culture/tradition. Kilbridem Suda & Njeru (2001) state that "a growing result of HIV infection in Kenya today is the increased burden and stress for the extended family, especially grandparents, who are left to care for AIDS orphans" (p. 29). They further state that HIV is eroding the traditional strengths of the extended family that had served in the past as an effective safety net. As can be noted with the number of nonrelatives who were care receivers, caregiving, which was traditionally a part of the microsystem is firmly embedded in the exosystem, where family, friends, and neighbors reside. This has implications for an approach to treatment that respects the differences between relative and non-relative caregivers. It may also have implications in the way that they carry out their roles.

Role Theory

Role theory focuses attention on "the stresses placed on the individual by the necessity to perform multiple roles, and the ways in which the interaction between persons is structured by their role expectations of one another and of themselves in their complementary positions; and the ways in which an individual's sense of self is influenced by the various positions she occupies and the effectiveness with which she plays her role" (Turner, 1996, p. 583). Role situations will probably result in interpersonal stress and/or interpersonal difficulties when there is conflict, ambiguity, strain and/or overload.

At this time in the social work profession, when there seems to be considerable emphasis on treating the person (or persons), it is all too easy to forget the depth at which problems begin. Many times, caregivers are in situations due to the positions they have been born into or otherwise achieved through no choice of their own, and they have been denied access to the resources that others, who are more fortunate, have in abundance. The use of role theory directs individuals away from excessive concern with individual psychopathology and toward an understanding of the social determinants of such behavior.

Role theory is used by other theories such as the problem solving theory and the life model, and it helps us understand the degree to which concerns may evolve because the caregiver in the family has received incomplete or inadequate socialization in the care giving role or not received sufficient support for the roles expected of them. Davis (1996) suggests "the concepts of role theory help focus our attention on the relationship between position, status, and access to resources and power" (p. 590). Kahn, Wolfe, Quinn, Snoek, and Rosenthal (1964) emphasize that roles are the result of expectations of others about appropriate behavior in a particular position. Concepts, central to role theory, that provide direction for framing the concept of burden include role conflict, overload, ambiguity, and changes in role expectations (University of Iowa, 2011). Role conflict is defined as psychological tension that is aroused by conflicting role pressures. Role conflict takes place when the individual experiences difficulty in performing his or her roles. "The demands may not be compatible to his/her role." (Turner, 1996, p. 583). Role ambiguity occurs when "roles expectations are unclear. Role ambiguity takes place when roles are developing or in the process of being redefined" (Turner, 1996, p. 583). Role overload develops when "a person is faced with complex roles. "Some individuals are able to balance family and work, while others experience stress" (Turner, 1996, p. 583).

Gender roles become internalized in personality traits as a result of powerful gender role socialization during childhood. Gender differences in sensitivity to relationships, role behaviors meaning, and use of social supports are expected to occur throughout the life cycle creating gender linked vulnerabilities that predispose women to experience greater distress (Epstein, 1995).

Ecological and role theories help to understand the challenges that caregivers face through placing value on the environmental influences of quality caregiving. When the family is unable to meet its traditional role of caregiving, the care is pushed outward toward friends and neighbors. For relatives who are caregivers, they too must rely upon the resources outside of the microsystem to meet the need for emotional and instrumental support. Equally important, is the macro system, which drives the feelings of stigma and discrimination that fuels the caregivers' inability to meet the responsibilities of care. The advocacy is directed largely at the macro system. The chronosystem helps to understand the socio-historical role of family within the context of the HIV/AIDS pandemic in Kenya. This operates at individual and community levels.

Role theory is equally important in understanding the unique impact of caregiving on women. Also, it contributes to an increased appreciation of the multiple roles that caregivers must master to be effective in the care assignment.

Most of the participants in the study were married or had children. Thus, their role as caregiver is not their own responsibility. Unfortunately, many are not financially secure in their ability to meet the needs of their own families, and the added role of caregiver can result in added stress.

Chapter 7

VIEWS FROM FAITH BASED AND NON GOVERNMENTAL ORGANIZATIONS

As noted in the study methods section, the team held two separate discussion forums with selected FBOs and NGOs. Caregivers and FBO/NGOs identified many of the same barriers. The factors and obstacles are associated with one of the four following factors: (1) Social-economic, (2) political strategy, (3) cultural, and (4) service coordination and implementation. Table 9 provides this detail.

Social-Economic Factors

"It is widely accepted that HIV/AIDS has major economic and social impacts on individuals, families, communities, and on society as a whole" (NACC, 2005, pg. 6). In Kenya, HIV/AIDS stagnates economic growth and development. The epidemic is negatively affecting an individual's health, lifespan, and productive capacity. There is a severe limitation on the increase of "human capacity," and its transfer between generations – numerous families are unable to pass on wealth to their children (NACC, 2005). The direct cost and social problems associated with caring for HIV/AIDS patients place significant strain on the entire society. HIV/AIDS is undermining development across all sectors of Kenya's economy and society (DFID, 2004).

Table 9:   Identified Factors and Obstacles

FACTORS	OBSTACLES
SOCIAL-ECONOMIC	High poverty levels Unemployment Faith Based Groups overburdened by the responsibility of caring Caregiver financial strain of providing care Negative cultural, social, economic and religious ideologies and practices. People living with HIV/AIDS still stigmatized.
POLITICAL STRATEGY	Political interference in program activities at the constituency level. Leadership disputes with Community Based Organizations Large NGOs not willing to share resources with small CBOs and Civil Society Organizations Conflict of roles and interest within Constituency AIDS Control Committees Mistrust, competition, suspicion and unwillingness to share information among different groups at various levels.
CULTURAL	Cultural norms that governed sexual behavior have been lost due to modernization. Polygamy was common; however, adultery was seriously frowned upon Marriage is delayed as there is a prolonged period of adolescence in order to finish school or train for a career. Although there were cultural norms that were considered to be harmful, many were believed to be important in establishing responsible adult behavior. There is a "sexual license" based on a poorly understood western sexual mores as seen on television etc.
SERVICE COORDINATION & IMPLEMENTATION	Poor coordination of program activities at the community level, including poor financial tracking. Target groups not involved in program planning and implementation Inadequate institutional capacity of implanting agencies. Transport sector not adequately involved in HIV/AIDS activities Duplication of activities and wastage of resources. Poor geographic coverage of interventions due to vastness of some regions.

(FBO and NGO Discussion Forums; NACC, 2005; KEC, 2000)

KEC (2000) asserts that poverty fuels the HIV/AIDS epidemic in numerous ways as identified below:

- Poor nutrition leads to great susceptibility to all illnesses.
- Poorly treated or untreated STDs due to the collapse of health services in poor countries.
- Engagement in commercial sex to make ends meet.
- Inability to get access to accurate information and being totally dependent on unscrupulous adverts which are suggestive without being informative.

(pg. 49)

The impact of the AIDS epidemic on these societies will be felt most strongly in the course of the next ten years. The social and economic consequences are already being widely felt, not only in the health, education, industry, and human resource sectors but also on the economy in general (Advert, 2009).

Political

According to NACC (2005), there have been challenges in the implementation of a national strategic plan both conceptually and practically. Kenya's National Strategic Plan is jointly owned by all stakeholders. This poses complications as it is essential that there is clear authority; however, it is difficult to establish this authority equitably. Previous attempts to develop national strategies have generally focused on interventions closest to the agency developing the plan, which have hindered implementation of a multi-sectoral approach. The Kenya National AIDS Strategic Plan emphasizes that each sector must have an understanding of how HIV/AIDS affects its work and how the epidemic is negatively impacting its sector.

Often limited definitions of roles and responsibilities undermine effective programmatic system performance. Contributing factors are often:

- Insufficient dissemination of policies;
- Absence of strategy to guide the system;
- Limited clarity on roles of structures and funding in relation to supporting the program;
- Inadequate understanding of service roles and responsibilities; and
- Limited knowledge regarding traditions and culture.

Leadership, direction, and support are major contributors to successful system performance. Inadequate coordination between key leadership is also a problem.

Cultural Practices

Kenya Episcopal Conference (KEC) (2000) asserts, "Despite accusation and counteraccusations, the fact is that the spread of HIV/AIDS has been fueled by the breakdown of morals" (pg. 45). Most religions uphold "sexual morality" as expressed by fidelity for the married and abstinence for the single. There are some members in religions that choose not to live up to the expressed ideals – these members have been identified as wishing to "have their cake and eat it too." They are choosing to use the façade of respectability offered by the religion at the same time breaking the tenets (KEC. 2000).

There are practices and beliefs that are affecting the spread of HIV/AIDS. Examples include: communal circumcision with one knife, ritual tattooing, and ear piercing. If these rituals are practiced, instruments must be properly sterilized (KEC, 2000). Also, the practice of widow inheritance has profound significance in various communities, often helping maintain clan identities. This practice during the era of HIV/AIDS has contributed to the spread of the disease. Assuming that a person is free from infections has often led to tragic consequences.

Chapter 8

THE WAY FORWARD: RECOMMENDATIONS

Family and informal caregivers are important members of the caregiving team. As the nation continues to advance in treatment of HIV and AIDS, it is important to develop the skills of caregivers and to provide them with needed recognition and social and instrumental support. Based on the HIV/AIDS Caregiver Focus Group participant feedback and the FBO/NGO discussion forums, themes were identified that led to the author's recommendations concerning support for caregivers and the patients that they serve.

Information, communication, and education interventions must go beyond raising awareness of HIV/AIDS. The recommendations are broken down into two areas: 1) Direct Support to Caregivers; and 2) Community-Based Support for Patients and their Families.

Recommendations Related to Direct Support to Caregivers

Recommendation 1: Increase financial support to caregivers

Although caregivers are often highly motivated to provide support, they often spoke about the lack of needed resources to provide food, clothing, transportation fares, and other supports. Often, the caregivers must use their own scarce resources. An option to direct financial support is access to resources that assists them in their caregiving role such as providing vouchers that can be used to make purchases. Caregivers should not have to go "empty handed" where there is food deprivation. Clearly, the recommendation includes systems of accountability to ensure the resources are used as intended.

Recommendation 2: Provide needed supplies to protect caregivers from infection

Caregivers do not have the needed supplies such as First Aid kits, antiseptics, towels, basins, soap, detergent, and gloves to safeguard their health. FBOs and NGOs could be helpful in collecting and disseminating these supplies.

Recommendation 3: Strengthen caregiving training

Caregivers are thrust into their role as caregivers, and it appears that they want training that will maximize the quality of the care that they deliver. They need training that focuses on effective practice with patients that are in denial. The caregivers recognize that the patients are not getting the maximum care if they are unable to accept their condition. The following areas need special attention as a training curriculum is developed or strengthened.

- *Targeted training on addressing the needs of children impacted by a parent with HIV/AIDS.*
  Caregivers indicated the stigma and discrimination that is uniquely visited upon children whose parents are infected. Caregivers expressed compassion for them; however, they may lack the skills to effectively address the mental health and well-being needs of the children, who are suffering from the multiple losses—including the loss of their childhood.
- *Skill-based training in working with persons in denial.*
  Caregivers expressed strong views about the challenges in providing the needed help to persons who denied their condition. It appears that they could benefit from strategies that help them to build the person's acceptance and willingness to receive needed treatment and care. Mosack & Petroll (2009) document that informal caregivers can help to make patients become more compliant.
- *Techniques to eliminate safety risks*

Caregivers seem to understand their needs to work in a safe environment. It is good practice to continuously reinforce safe practices and to ensure that they are being followed.

- *Targeted training to youth caregivers*
  Unfortunately, the HIV/AIDS pandemic calls into service the young and the old. It is recommended that specialized training be provided to young caregivers. Giving Hope Empowerment is an example of a program that exists and is being implemented by some organizations in Kenya. This program should be expanded.
- *Specific training in ethics of caregiving and end of life care*
  Caregivers voiced concerns about ethical dilemmas, especially regarding end of life care. Targeted training on ethics, spirituality, and end of life care could assist them in addressing situations when they are in conflict related to confidences.

Recommendation 4: Strengthen emphasis on self-care

Caregiving literature is replete with data that documents the wear and tear that caregiving can have. To address these stressors and possible risks to mental health, it is recommended that caregivers invest in self-care. It appears that support groups are one means of such care, and there may be other strategies that FBOs and NGOs could introduce to caregivers to ensure that they maintained their positive health and outlook.

Recommendations for Community-Based Organizations

Recommendation 5: Increase Knowledge Regarding HIV/AIDS

Caregivers noted that the spread of HIV/AIDS continues because individuals under their care did not fully understand all aspects of the disease. Although there has been a reduction in the number of cases, there still continues to be the need to have strategies to increase public awareness related to prevention, treatment, and caregiving.

- Provide HIV/AIDS education to the infected and affected in the community for self-dependence.
- Offer HIV/AIDS training to the affected, particularly Home-based Caregivers.
- Promote Safe Sexual Behavior

    - Promoting abstinence before marriage is paramount among both youth and adults.
    - Development and implementation of behavior interventions with an emphasis on greater condom use among sex workers.
    - Encouraging faithfulness among married couples.

- Encourage HIV Testing

    - Encourage HIV/AIDS testing among sexually active youth and adult risk groups.
    - Provide community based health services facilities with HIV/AIDS test kits and funding to expand ability to provide testing.

- Provide community awareness regarding the negative impact of stigmatism and discrimination among HIV/AIDS patients and their caregivers. This awareness should also include targeted strategies identified using grass-roots techniques.
- Provided targeted campaigns for women that address gender discrimination in treatment—a human rights campaign for women.
- Provide targeted campaigns and training for youth caregivers. Models such as "Giving Hope Empowerment" are active in several organizations in Kenya (Church World Service, 2008).

Recommendation 6: Increase Available AIDS Treatment

Availability, affordability, and accessibility are important to the treatment of AIDS. Caregivers and community-based organizations support the need for treatment to be available to all aspects of the community.

Recommendation 7: Provide HIV/AIDS patients with medical support and food supplements

Food deprivation and lack of medical support remain barriers to effectively addressing HIV and AIDS. The community level planning should address these serious deficiencies and create the needed linkages and support systems.

Recommendation 8: Advocate for the Development and Implementation of Community Based Programs

There is a consensus among stakeholders that the best approach to stemming HIV/AIDS is one that engages every layer of the community, including government, nongovernmental units, faith-based organizations, churches and other places of worship, and families, who live with the impact of HIV/AIDS. Home-based care is essential, and it is needed to maximize quality of life. For it to be effective, partnerships are needed.

- Encourage partnership between FBOs and NGOs to provide holistic home-based care to HIV/AIDS patients and their caregivers, including both medical/clinic and community/development components.
- Programs for relatives and extended family that emphasize the need for them to step in to prevent children from becoming orphans
- Community-based caregiver recognition and appreciation ceremonies are also important to bring attention to the important role of caregivers in Kenya.

Recommendation 9: Develop and train organizations on professional standards for practice with family and informal caregivers.

The National Association of Social Workers (2010) provides examples of such standards that specifically address 1) ethics and values, 2) qualifications, 3) knowledge, 4) cultural and linguistic competence, 5) assessment, 6) service planning, delivery, and monitoring; 7) advocacy, 8) collaboration, 9) practice, evaluation, and improvement; 10) documentation, 11) workload, and 12) professional development and competence.

Recommendation 10: Engage in more community-based participatory research related to caregiving.

There is inadequate Kenya-specific research on caregiving. A review of the literature documents the dearth of research. Using the support of Schools of Social Work and organizations serving them, the community can be served well by developing its own research agenda that examines more closely areas that are important at the community level. Gysels, Pell, Straus & Pool (2011) assert that End of Life Care (EOL) in sub-Saharan Africa lacks a sound evidence-base to develop effective and appropriate services.

These ten recommendations build upon the 2010 targets set in the Kenya's National HIV and AIDS Strategic Plan in that they include specific focus on how HIV is affecting specific groups, social and economic inequalities, stigma and discrimination, and the need for sources of money to support demand for antiretroviral drugs and needed supplies. The recommendations also support the need to address the erosion of the traditional extended family care network that has historically served as protective factors for children, old people, individuals with disabilities, and other vulnerable groups in need of protection and care.

In closing the caregivers have voiced their concerns, and they provide increased understanding of their needs. We end this book with the powerful voice of a caregiver, who reminds us that caregiving is a shared responsibility.

> We as caregivers...most of us finding ourselves as caregivers was not out of our own liking, we did not start as caregivers, but we found ourselves in a situation that we were taking care of these people because we are caught up in the circumstances with them – although we help and assist them, at time we are stranded on what to do because we are not trained to keep them well and assist them well, but it has become our responsibility to help them.

Harambee!

Appendices

APPENDIX I
MISSIONARY VOICES

Heart of God –Kenya

After more than 30 years of marriage, Mike and Pat Heiser left their family to share the love of Jesus. Moving 9000 miles to Meru, Kenya has changed their lives. They founded Heart of God – Kenya, developing the following Confession for the ministry:

We have and operate in the blessings of Abraham
The leadership skills of David
The wisdom of Solomon. And the strength of Samson
The revelation of Paul
The servant-hood of Jesus
The love of God
And the anointing of the Holy Spirit
We walk in divine health
God's prosperity and wealth
And the wisdom of God
We're blessed to be a blessing
To all we encounter
Amen

(Heart of God Kenya, 2010)

Mike and Pat share the following stories of the lives of the children that they have adopted. Their ministries have touched the hearts of many.

Tossed from family to family, Ken survived the last five years by proving his value. When His parents died of AIDS and his older brothers were scattered, Ken became the village's stray dog that no one really wanted. When Jonah (oldest boy) went to visit his village in 2007, he saw how his little brother Ken was exploding with anger and extremely rebellious so Jonah asked if he could bring him home.

Ken's eyes got as big as saucers as he saw all the cars, trucks, and shops in Meru. Ken had entered another world. Everything was so different from his mud-hutted village. The first time his anger exploded, he ran, but this time he got lost amidst all the crowds and traffic of Meru. Mike found him bewildered and ready to come home. Since then, Ken has gradually calmed down and settled into the routine of family life. Ken enjoys school and is quickly catching up. Yes, he is still highly competitive and explosive at times, but the promise that "love never fails" (I Corinthians 13:8) has once again proven the faithfulness of God's Word." (Ken's parents died from AIDS)

JONAH: In 2003, Mike bought Jonah for $3. His parents both died when he was only 5 years old. His uncle *sold* Jonah and his brother to different people. First Jonah worked on a man's shamba (farm). Then he worked as a water boy in Meru's market. Mike bought (yes, money was given for his freedom) Jonah from the market and brought him home. Quickly Jonah excelled in school, soccer, and everything. Even his clothes and bed were the neatest! Soon however we discovered that Jonah was trying to be first, so we would value him. Slowly he is learning that God loves him and so do we- no matter what. This year 2009, Jonah has returned to the Market to share the GOOD NEWS with some of the same people he used to run wild with. These boys have watched Jonah being transformed from a street boy to a very confident young man whom they eagerly listen to as he shares the GOOD NEWS with them because if Jesus can change Jonah, perhaps there is hope for them too!" (Jonah's parents died from AIDS)

Moses is our fire king! We cook outside, and usually Moses is the one manning the fire. He blows on the coals, and they come alive! Even away from the fire, he lights up the place with his contagious smile. However, those first few months after Moses joined our family in October 2004 were horrible. Moses constantly cursed 24/7. Many times he ran back to his mama, who had attempted to kill him with a machete'. If there had been any other place for him, we would have gladly surrendered custody. However, we were committed to providing a safe place for him. One day his mouth was so vulgar that we tried reasoning with him, but Moses would not listen and attempted to run away again. However, this time Mike caught him. Moses kicked and screamed, but Mike just held him tight. Finally after almost an hour Moses started crying like a baby, and Mike begun rocking him. The war was over!!

Apoche ran to the street when life with her crippled grandmother and insane mama became overwhelming. She discovered that street life was difficult too. Would the missionaries give her a fresh start and be willing to open their home to someone like her, who had done so many bad things? We did! Watching her has been like watching an ugly worm transform into a beautiful butterfly. Now she is born again and delivered from AIDS! Apoche is from the Turkana tribe. She has been with us since February 2006. She is in 7th grade. Fewer than 5% of the Turkana tribe can read or write, but Apoche is fluent in both Swahili and English. She has a tremendous gift of leadership and is quite helpful with our 10 younger boys. Apoche will graduate from NEEMA Bible College in August 2010 and primary school in 2011. She hopes to return to her people and teach them to read but more importantly to share the unconditional love of God, which has set her free."

Trees of Healing

Trees Of Healing, Inc., (TOH) mission's work in East Africa was founded in 2001 by the current Executive Director, Lynn Miller. There, she was touched by the destitute state of the people, especially the suffering of innocent women and children. Since the inception of the ministry, it has been one of TOH's daily activities to supply the people of Meru Central and Tharaka District support for their livelihood. The needs of the people of this semi-arid area are many because it is one of the most undeveloped, overlooked areas of Kenya. Meru/Tharaka has one of the highest prevalence rates of Aids in Kenya - in 2001 the prevalence rate was 38%.

In 2005, the organization registered a branch ministry called Hand of God in Kenya and that ministry, run by Kenya citizens, is currently working in Meru Town and Tharaka District implementing various projects, which include renovating and providing houses, food, clothing and schooling for families with HIV/AIDS, street children, and other destitute families; micro-financing small businesses; working with communities to supply clean, safe drinking water, and initiating projects that provide jobs for the local people.

Lynn Miller asserts,

"God spoke to me while I was ministering to women in prison and street children. He told me to start a ministry for these that had lost all hope of ever having their dreams or destinies fulfilled. He told me to call the ministry HAND OF GOD MINISTRY KENYA because truly it will take His hand of provision to help these people."

As the founder of TOH, she has written short articles regarding particular topics related to her missionary work in Kenya as illustrated below.

HIV/AIDS Pandemic

If God is close to the poor — and if we want to be close to God — Jeremiah shows us how it is done. We can be close to God by being close to the poor. We can have intimacy with the Lord by caring about what he cares about. Isaiah says of God, "He is determined that the poor of his people will find refuge" (Isaiah 14:32). Again, note the Lord's resolve: he isn't just hoping, wondering, longing, and wishing — he is determined. God will find a way for the poor to find refuge. And for us, being close to God requires that we share in his determination.

Tharaka Clinic

Healthcare is neither easily accessible nor affordable for many Kenyans living in these rural villages. Poverty creates a large barrier to the acquisition of healthcare in general, but in rural areas in particular. Most of the locals in the Tharaka area cannot afford consultation, treatment, or pharmacy fees. Nor can they afford transport to clinics and hospitals located in the towns. The combined cost of transport and consultation is more than seven times what many people earn in a day. Malaria, typhoid, diarrhea, measles, tetanus, pneumonia, and malnutrition are preventable and treatable, and yet they kill thousands of people every year. Addressing the health care needs in the villages is vital to improving living conditions. Our long-term goals include decreasing child mortality in the region; improving women's health; offering pre- and post-natal care; and to provide treatment for people with HIV/AIDS, malaria, typhoid, gastroenteritis, and other endemic illnesses. We also hope to expand to include a small surgery suite and an in-patient ward. The more treatment we can provide and procedures we are equipped to handle, the more lives we save.

APPENDIX II
INTERNATIONAL FEDERATION OF SOCIAL WORKERS: HISTORICAL PERSONS

The IFSW has acknowledged the following social workers for their dedication and accomplishments regarding international programs, services and advocacy.

Alice Salomon (1872-1948)

Alice Salomon is one of the principal founders of professional social work in Germany and the creator of German social work education. As a young social reformer and feminist leader in 1893, she helped establish the Girls' and Women's Groups for Social Aid Work, and in 1899 she cofounded the first one-year course in vocational welfare training, which in 1908 became a two-year training program. She was a leader in the development of social work as a profession for women and for men before, during, and after World War I. She led the efforts to restore the nation after the war and fought the Nazi movement until being forced to emigrate in 1937. A leading German school of social work in Berlin bears her name. (The Social Work Dictionary, Robert L. Barker, NASW Press)

Jane M. Hoey (1892-1968)

Jane M. Hoey's major contribution to social work was in the establishment and enforcement of standards in public welfare administration. The daughter of Irish immigrants, she was born in Greeley County, Nebraska, USA. After receiving an MA in political science from Colombia University and a diploma from the New York School of Philanthropy in 1916, she began working for Harry Hopkins at the New York Board of Child Welfare. Employed by the American Red Cross, she later became secretary of the Bronx Committee of the New York Tuberculosis and Health Association. She helped organize the Health Division of the New York Welfare Council and became its assistant director in 1926. A combination of family and administrative experience helped acquaint her with the political world. Her political skills were helpful in negotiations with US government officials and in program interpretation when she served as a delegate to the United Nations. Jane M. Hoey later became the director of social research for the National Tuberculosis Association and served as president of the National Conference of Social Work, the Council on Social Work Education, and the William J. Kerby Foundation. The Jane M. Hoey Chair in Social Policy was established by the Colombia University School of Social Work. Between 1931 and 1953, Hoey published a number of articles related to government policy and welfare. Larraine M. Edwards Jane M. Hoey bequeathed some of her fortune to IFSW. The money was put into a Solidarity Fund, which is used to provide support for social work development in poorer countries or facilitate participation in IFSW Conferences for social workers from target countries. At IFSW World and Regional Conferences, a Jane Hoey Fund Auction is always held to raise funds for IFSW's solidarity work.

Andrew Mouravieff-Apostol (1913-2001)

Dr. Andrew Mouravieff-Apostol, known to the international social work community as Andy, was born in Cannes, France on 7th February 1913 of Russian/Ukrainian parents. His father served as a diplomat but gave up his career on his marriage to Andy's mother in order to manage her vast estates in Ukraine. They were in England when the war broke out and soon afterwards they founded a hospital in London for British Officers.

The 1917 Revolution made it impossible for aristocrats like the Mouravieff-Apostols to return to Russia, and it was not until the time of the Perestroika in the 1980s, that Andy was able to visit his beloved home country again. Because of all the care and assistance his family had given his compatriots before, during, and after the Revolution, he was warmly received and he also was awarded an Honoris Causa Doctorate by one of the Universities in the former Soviet Union. Andy started his career as a journalist and foreign correspondent in England for the Daily Telegraph and Evening Standard before and during World War II. He also served in the Free French military forces during the war.

After the war and on the direct encouragement of Winston Churchill, Andy left journalism and took up a position with the World Council of Churches and later with the United Nations High Commissioner for Refugees. He worked in a number of countries with resettlement programs, mainly in South America. In Brazil, he met his future wife Ellen and the couple settled in Geneva. Andy also worked as a professional interpreter at the United Nations and other international bodies. Andy was a talented linguist, speaking 6-7 languages from which he was able to interpret into English.

From 1975 to 1992, Andy was IFSW Secretary General, and he was elected lifelong Honorary President in 1992. For IFSW, Andy was the cornerstone. He communicated with social workers of all countries with warmth, knowledge and diplomacy and became like a father for the international social work community. At IFSW General Meetings/World Conferences, starting in 2004, in memory of Andrew Mouravieff-Apostol, a medal with an accompanying diploma shall be presented to an individual or organization that over time has made a significant contribution to international social work.

Litsa Alexandraki (1918-1984)

Litsa Alexandraki was born in Russia to Greek parents in 1918. She graduated from the Faculty of Law at Athens University in June 1940 and seconded as a lawyer by the Areos Pagos (High Court) to the First Instance Court of Athens in August 1941. During the Second World War,

Litsa Alexandraki worked as voluntary nurse (Graduate of the School of Voluntary Nurses, Greek Red Cross) in Greece and was appointed several times during the war to high and responsible positions by the Swiss, Greek, and International Red Cross Committees.

From 1946-1950 she studied criminology, sociology, psychology, social work, and education at the London School of Economics and at the University of London. Upon her return from England, she was appointed Advisor to the Ministry of Welfare in Greece. She initiated a program to assist the families whose heads had been killed in the war or separated from the families for other reasons. She participated in a number of law drafting committees, assisted in the reorganization of the schools of social work, and taught social work. Litsa Alexandraki was the founder of the Hellenic Association of Social Workers and was three times elected as President of the International Federation of Social Workers. She served in this position from 1962 to1968. During this time, she expanded the IFSW membership to Asia, Africa, and Latin America. When Litsa Alexandraki resigned as IFSW President in 1968, she became Honorary President until her death in 1984. An international award for outstanding social work was introduced in her name in 1988. It was given to Andrew and Ellen Mouravieff Apostol in 1992 for their long and faithful work for IFSW as Secretary General and Associate Secretary General, respectively.

Celia B. Weisman (1918-2000)

Dr. Celia Bach Weisman was the IFSW Main Representative to the UN New York for 12 years (1988-2000). The daughter of an orthodox rabbi, she was born in London and later accompanied her family to the United States at an early age. After receiving the baccalaureate degree, she began teaching the German language. She earned her master of social work degree from the University of Pittsburgh after learning about anti-Semitism and committing herself to its demise. She earned her doctorate in social work from Columbia University at age fifty. She worked passionately and energetically in support of social justice throughout her life. She held a faculty position at the Wurzweiler School of Social Work where her areas of specialization were gerontology and group work. She lectured nationally and internationally. Knowledgeable about the social work profession's strong traditions around social development and advocacy in the local, regional, national and international arenas for policy and action, Celia worked quite tirelessly to perpetuate these efforts in meeting our contemporary needs. She very effectively organized the annual Social Work Day at the United Nations, attracting audiences filled with professional social workers and social work students, eager to undertake their roles in transmitting knowledge about the human condition, in influencing decision-makers, and in contributing to the development of knowledge through research.

Celia participated in the Executive Committee meetings of IFSW, reporting regularly on the key issues and recommending policy positions, both during the meetings and through the IFSW Newsletter. Active also in the New York City Chapter of the National Association of Social Workers, Celia made many contributions to their International Committee.

Mary E. Richmond (1861-1928)

Considered one of the principal founders of professional social work, Mary E. Richmond led the Charity Organization Societies (COSs) movement to develop schools to train social caseworkers. She taught volunteers and paid employees in various settings and developed some of the first teaching programs for social work.

Eileen McGowan Kelly (1946-1996)

Eileen McGowan Kelly was the Director of Peace and International Affairs for the National Association of Social

Workers, USA. During her tenure at NASW, she worked tirelessly as an international leader, promoting international social work and peace and advocating for human rights. She was born in North Attleboro, Massachusetts, held dual Masters Degrees in rehabilitation counseling (George Washington University) and social work (Catholic University). Her extensive professional history included administrative responsibilities, policy and program development, legislative and community advocacy, and consultations worldwide. She also served on the boards of a number of social service organizations including PeaceLinks and the US Committee - International Conference on Social Welfare.

Eileen McGowan Kelly was known for her tremendous accomplishments advancing the social work profession's role in the international arena. Eileen's vision was to promote international links and exchanges for professional social workers and social work associations throughout the world. Realizing the global impact of social issues and the significant role of social workers, Eileen worked with intense passion and commitment to link social workers throughout the world with another.

Mary Stewart (1862/3– 1925)

Mary Stewart, who in 1895 became the first almoner in the United Kingdom, was a trained Charity Organization Society worker, experienced in assessing needs and accessing resources - skills still required. A woman of tact, compassion, and quiet determination, she gradually overcame the suspicions of the medical staff. Assistants were appointed; volunteer helpers came forward. The experiment proved successful and cost effective. By 1903 almoners, including one man, had been appointed to discuss the problems and possibilities of the work and for mutual support, forming the Hospital Almoners Committee - the first professional social work association and the forerunner of the British Association of Social Workers (BASW).

Eileen Younghusband (1902-1981)

Author, educator, and a major organizer of British social work, Dame Eileen was on the faculty of the London School of Economics for many years. She helped establish Great Britain's Citizen's Advice Bureaus (CABs) during World War II and the modern British juvenile court system, and she redeveloped the International Association of Schools of Social Work (IASSW). Her classic social work texts include Social Work and Social Change (1964) and Casework with Families and Children (1965).

Rene Sand (1877-1953)

Dr. Rene Sand became a social lighthouse for the guidance of those professionally engaged in medical or social work; he was above all a humanist, actively concerned with the society of his time.

He was born at Ixelles, Brussels, Belgium, on 30th January 1877 of Luxembourg and French blood, but had Belgian nationality. In 1900 he became a doctor of medicine, and as a doctor he brought together his concern for medical research, education, health, and social protection. As Secretary General of the Red Cross in Belgium, he was one of the promoters of social work, and it was on his initiative that the Belgian National Committee of Social Work was set up in 1948. Dr. Sand took a very active part in the International Conference of Social Work (now International Council on Social Welfare), ICSW. The organization later founded the Rene Sand prize in his memory. The prize is presented every two years to persons or organizations that, in their work for social development, have best contributed to the promotion of social welfare.

(From "Rene Sand and the Culture of Human Values" by Alain Anciaux, ICSW)

Jane Addams (1860-1935)

Jane Addams won worldwide recognition in the first third of the 20th Century as a pioneer social worker, feminist, and internationalist. Born in Cedarville, Illinois, USA she started studying medicine but gave it up due to poor health. In the late 1880s, she visited Toynbee Hall in London's East End and was inspired to go back to Chicago and open a similar house. In 1889, she opened Hull-House in an effort to help families, take care of children, nurse the sick, and listen to troubled people. By its second year, Hull-House was host to more than 2,000 people every week. The House developed by also opening an employment bureau, an art gallery, a public kitchen, a library, and music and drama schools.

As her reputation grew, Jane Addams was drawn into larger fields of civic responsibilities as the Chicago Board of Education and later as President of the National Conference on Charities and Corrections (later the National Conference of Social Work). She was the first woman to receive an honorary degree by Yale University. Publishing about women's rights and peace, she became President of the Women's International League for Peace and Freedom, which still is an active international NGO. Addams urged the United States to join the League of Nations and the World Court. Jane Addams was awarded the Nobel Peace Prize in 1931. At the award ceremony, the Norwegian Nobel Committee paid tribute to Jane Addams by stating:

"She held fast to the ideal of peace even during the difficult hours when other considerations and interests obscured it from her compatriots and drove them into conflict."

ABOUT THE AUTHORS

Dr. Charnetta Gadling-Cole is an Assistant Professor at the University of Alabama at Birmingham (UAB) in the College of Arts and Sciences, Department of Social Work. She holds secondary appointments as a Scientist in the UAB Center for Aging and UAB Center for AIDS Research. She is also a scholar in the UAB Minority Health and Health Disparities Research Center and there Geriatrics Education Center. Dr. Gadling-Cole's research interests are in the areas of geriatrics/gerontology, caregiving, and international social work.

Dr. Sandra Edmonds Crewe is a Professor and Associate Dean for the Howard University School of Social Work. She also serves on the faculty of the Howard University graduate school. Dr. Crewe is the director of the Multidisciplinary Center for Gerontology. Her research interests are in the areas of aging, caregiving, and kinship care.

Professor Mildred C. Joyner retired as Chair of the Undergraduate Social Work Department at West Chester University after more than 30 years of service. Professor Joyner currently serves as the President of the Council on Social Work Education. She is equally a member of the CSWE Gero-Ed Center (gerontological education) and the National Association of Social Workers. Her research interests include child abuse, diversity issues, and gerontology.

REFERENCES

AIDS.Gov (2011). A Timeline of AIDS. Retrieved from http://www.aids.gov/hiv-aids-basics/hiv-aids-101/overview/aids-timeline/

African Council of Aids Service Organization (2009). Retrieved from http://www.africaso.net/index.php?option=com_content&task=view&id=39&Itemid=48

Avert (2011). AIDS Timeline. Retrieved from http://www.avert.org/aids-timeline.htm

Avert (2009). HIV and AIDS in Africa. Retrieve from http://www.avert.org/hiv-aids-africa.htm.

AVERT (2010). President Emergency Plan for AIDS Relief (PEPFAR). Retrieved from http://www.avert.org/pep far.htm

Barretta-Herman, A. (2005) 'A Reanalysis of the IASSW World Census 2000', *International Social Work* 48(6): 794–808.

BBS (2011). Kenya Country Profile. Retrieved from http://news.bbc.co.uk/2/hi/africa/country_profiles/1024563.st m).

Board on International Scientific Organizations (BISO) (2008). International Collaborations in Behavioral and Social Sciences Research: Report of a Workshop. http://www.nap.edu/openbook.php?record_id=12053&page=20

Brown, A. W., Gourdine, R.M. & Crewe, S.E. (2011). Inabel Burns Lindsay: Social Work Pioneer Contributor to Practice and Education through a Socio-cultural Perspective. *Journal of Sociology and Social Welfare.*

Brofenbrenner's Ecological Model (2011). Retrieved from http://www.bing.com/images/search?q=Ecological+syst ems+theory&view=detail&id=8F23909D6AD44EAAA B3E38F66DB8290AD099AFDF&first=121&FORM=I DFRIR

Cichocki, M. (2009). The History of HIV/AIDS the Birth of the Protease Inhibitor. about.com Guide, http://aids. about.com/od/newlydiagnosed/a/hivtimeline_2.htm

Churches in Kenya, (2010). http://www.kenyaspace.com/ churchesinkenya.htm

Council on Social Work Education(2010). Commission on Global Education. http://www.cswe.org/About/govern ance/CommissionsCouncils/15555.aspx

Council on Social Work Education, (2010). Katherine A. Kendall Institute http://www.cswe.org/CentersInitia tives/16764.aspx

Crewe, S. E., & Stowell-Ritter, A. (2003, November). *Grandparents raising grandchildren in the District of Columbia: Focus group report.* Retrieved from AARP, Knowledge Management. Retrieved from http://assets. aarp.org/rgcenter/general/dc_gp.pdf

Crewe, S.E., Brown, A.W., & Gourdine, R.M. (2008). Inabel Burns Lindsay: A social worker, educator, and administrator uncompromising in the pursuit of social justice or all. *Affilia* 23(4), 363-367.

Freshwater, D., Sherwood, G., Drury,V. Cowan, E. (2006).International research collaboration: Issues, benefits and challenges of the global network. Journal of Research in Nursing, vol.11. 4: 295-303.

Garber, R. (2000) 'Social Work and Globalization', *Canadian Social Work* 2(1) (Summer) 17 (Special Issue): 198–215.

Germain, C. B and Gitterman, A. (1995) , Ecological perspective. Encyclopdedia of Social Work pp. 816-824 NASW,Vol 1

Global Coalition on Women and AIDS (2009). *Support Women Caregiver: Fight AIDS. http://www.pacttz. org/pdfs/59.%20Support%20Women%20Caregivers%2 0Fight%20AIDS.pdf*

Gourdine, R.M., Crewe, S.E. & Brown, A.W. (2008). Building an institution second to none: Dr. Inabel Burns Lindsay—a social work leader in the academy. *Journal of Human Behavior in the Social Environment,* 18(3), 364-391.

Green, L, Fryer, G., Froom, P., Culpepper, L & Froom, J. (2004). Opportunities, Challenges, and Lessons of International Research in Practice-Based Research Networks: The Case of an International Study of Acute Otitis Media. *Annals of Family Medicine* 2:429-433.

Gysels, M., Pell, C., Straus, L. & Pool, R. (2011). End of life care in sub-Saharan Africa: A systematic review of qualitative literature. *BMC Palliative Care*, 10(6)

Haag (2009). NGOs and spatial dimensions of poverty in Kenya. African Studies Association UK Biennial Conference.

Healy, L (2008). Exploring the history of social work as a human rights profession, *International Social Work* 2008 51: 735

Hepworth, Rooney, & Larsen (1997). Direct social work practice: Theory and skills 5th edition. Brooks/Cole Publishing publishers

International Association of Schools of Social Work (2010). http://www.iasswaiets.org/index.php?option=com_conte nt&task=view&id=1&Itemid=1

International Federation of Social workers, (2010). Historical Persons. http://www.ifsw.org/p38001894.html

International Federation of Social Workers (2010) International Federation of Social Workers. Retrieved from http://www.ifsw.org/

The Non-Governmental Organizations Co-Ordination Act 1990 Kenya. Retrieved from http://www.usig.org/ countryinfo/laws/Kenya/Nongovernmental_Organizatio ns_Coordination_Act_1990__Kenya_%20.pdf

Kenya Episcopal Conference (KEC) (2006). Inventory of the Catholic Church Responses to HIV & AIDS in Kenya. Retrieved from http://kardsafrica.org/index/ images/pdf/aids_inventory_2006.pdf

Kenya Minister of Health (2005). Kenya National HIV/AIDS Strategic Plan

Kilbride, P., Sudoa, Collette, Njero, E. (2001) *Street children in Kenya: voices of children*. Westport, CT: Bergin and Garvey.

King, C.S. (1986). A Testament of Hope: The Essential Writings and Speeches of Martin Luther King, Jr. , New York: Harper Collins Publishers

Kipp, W., Tindyebwa, D., Karamagi, E., & Rubaale, T (2006). Family caregiving to AIDS patiesnts: the role of gender in caregiving burden in Uganda. *Journal of International Women's Studies* 7(4), pp. 1-13.

Mageto, P. (2005) silent church = death: a critical look at the church's response to HIV/AIDS. Currents in Theology and Mission.

Machyo, C. (2001) The Catholic Church and the HIV/AIDS Pandemic in Kenya: An Exploration of Issues. Retrieved from http://www.fiuc.org/iaup/esap/publications/cuea/eajourn1aidsch.php

Maps of the World (2011). Thika Maps. Retrieved from http://mapsof.net/thika

Maslow, Abraham H. "A Theory of Human Motivation." *Psychological Review* 50 (1943): 370-396.

Med.Net (2004). First public healthcare and HIV/AIDS programme in Kibera, Kenya. Retrieved from http://www.news-medical.net/news/2004/10/22/5757.aspx

Methodist Church in Kenya (2010). Retrieved from http://www.methodistchurchkenya.org/index.php?page=health-wholeness

Mike & Pat Heiser (2010) Kenyan News. Heart of God Newsletter

Mosack, K.E. & Petroll,A. (2009) Patients' perspecties on informal caregiver involvement in HIV health care appointments. *AIDS Patient Care STDS*, December 23(12), pp. 1043-1051.

Muchiri, J. (2002). HIV/AIDS, breaking the silence: a guide book for pastoral caregivers. Nairobi, Kenya : Paulines Publications Africa.

Muraah, W.M and Kiarie, W.N.2001. *HIV and AIDS, Facts that could change your Life*, English Press, Nairobi.

National AIDS Control Council (2005) Kenya National HIV/AIDS Strategic Plan. Retrieved from http://www.nacc.or.ke/2007/images/down loads/knasp_20052010_final_report.pdf

National AIDS and STI Control Program (NASCOP) (2005). AIDS in Kenya Trends, Interventions and Impact. http://www.aidskenya.org/public_site/webroot/ca che/article/file/AIDSinKenyaFinal.pdf

National AIDS and STI Control Program (NASCOP) (2002), National Home-Based Care Programme and Service Guidelines. Ministry of Health Nairobi, Kenya

National Association of Social Workers (2010). *NASW standards for social work practice with family caregivers of older adults*. NASW Press: Washington, DC.

National Association of Social Work - North Carolina Chapter: International Social Work; Retrieved from http://www.naswnc.org/displaycommon.cfm?an=1&sub articlenbr=51

Onyango R., (2008). Home-based Health Care (HBHC): Are Women Caregivers at Risk? A Study of Busia and Teso Districts in Western Kenya *Education for Health.* 22:1. Retrieved from: http://www.educationforhealth. net/

PACANET (2005). The Church's Role in Strengthening the Family in an Era of HIV/AIDS A Position Paper by the Pan-African Christian AIDS Network

PEPFAR (2009). Care for People Living with HIV/AIDS. Retrieved from http://www.pepfar.gov/press/84749.htm

Pirraglia , P. A; Bishop, D.; Herman, D.S.; Trisvan, E.; Lopez, R.A.; Torgersen, C.S., Van Hof, A.M.; Anderson, B.J.; Miller, I., and Stein, M.D. (2005), Caregiver burden and depression among informal caregivers of HIV-infected individuals. *Journal of General Internal Medicine,* 20(6), pp. 510-514.

SFA Partners (2010). A Prepared Place. http://www. standforafrica.org/Partners.htm

Softkenya,com (2011). Machakos County. Retrieved from http://softkenya.com/county/machakos-county/

Tearfund, (2006). Why Churches Can play a Crucial Role in tackling HIV and AIDS in Africa. Retrieved from http://www.crin.org/docs/tearfund_hiv.pdf

Trochim, W. (2006). Qualitative Approches. Retrieved from http://www.socialresearchmethods.net/kb/qualapp.php

The University of Iowa (2011). Family Involvement and Care Study. Retrieved from http://www.nursing.uiowa. edu/research/fic/theoretical.htm

Tutu, D. (1999). *No Future Without Forgiveness*. Image. ISBN 0-385-49690-7.

UNAIDS (2011). Support Women Caregivers: Fight AIDS. Retrieved from http://data.unaids.org/pub/FactSheet/ 2006/20060719_GCWA_FS_Support_Women_Caregiv ers_en.pdf

UNICEF, (2004). Children on the Brink. http:// www.unicef.org/publications/files/cob_layout6-013.pdf.

UNICEF, (2004). Girls, HIV/AIDS and Education. Retrieved from http://www.unicef.org/publications/files/ Girls_HIV_AIDS_and_Education_(English)_rev.pdf.

US Congress (2010). CHAPTER 83 - United States Leadership against HIV/AIDS, Tuberculosis and Malaria.

US State Department (2011). Background Note: Kenya. Retrieved from http://www.state.gov/r/pa/ei/bgn/2962. htm

U.S. Department of State (2008). 2008 Country Profile: Kenya. Retrieved from 2006-2009.pepfar.gov/press/ 81596.htm

WEMA Centre (2011). WEMA Centre Transforming Street Children. Retrieved from http://www.wemacentre.org/ thika/thika

World Bank (2011). World Bank and NGOs. Retrieved from http://library.duke.edu/research/subject/guides/ ngo_guide/igo_ngo_coop/ngo_wb.html

INDEX

www.ingramcontent.com/pod-product-compliance
Lightning Source LLC
Chambersburg PA
CBHW070923270326
41927CB00011B/2701